Data Interpretation Questions
in Paediatrics

Data Interpretation Questions
in Paediatrics

Fiona Finlay
Consultant Community Paediatrician
Child Health Department
Newbridge Hill
Bath, UK

Liz Lambert
Senior Registrar in Neonatology
Southampton General Hospital
Southampton, UK

Simon Lenton
Consultant Community Paediatrician
Child Health Department
Newbridge Hill
Bath, UK

Jacqui Clinch
Senior Registrar in Paediatrics
Southmeads Hospital
Bristol, UK

b

Blackwell
Science

© 1998 by
Blackwell Science Ltd
Editorial Offices:
Osney Mead, Oxford OX2 0EL
25 John Street, London WC1N 2BL
23 Ainslie Place, Edinburgh EH3 6AJ
350 Main Street, Malden
   MA 02148 5018, USA
54 University Street, Carlton
   Victoria 3053, Australia
10, rue Casimir Delavigne
   75006 Paris, France

Other Editorial Offices:

Blackwell Wissenschafts-Verlag GmbH
   Kurfürstendamm 57
   10707 Berlin, Germany

Blackwell Science KK
   MG Kodenmacho Building
   7–10 Kodenmacho Nihombashi
   Chuo-ku, Tokyo 104, Japan

First published 1998

Set by Setrite Typesetters,
Hong Kong

The Blackwell Science logo is a
trade mark of Blackwell Science Ltd,
registered at the United Kingdom
Trade Marks Registry

For further information on
Blackwell Science, visit our website:
www.blackwell-science.com

DISTRIBUTORS

Marston Book Services Ltd
PO Box 269
Abingdon, Oxon OX14 4YN
(*Orders*: Tel: 01235 465500
            Fax: 01235 465555)

USA
Blackwell Science, Inc.
Commerce Place
350 Main Street
Malden, MA 02148 5018
(*Orders*: Tel: 800 759 6102
                 781 388 8250
          Fax: 781 388 8255)

Canada
Login Brothers Book Company
324 Saulteaux Crescent
Winnipeg, Manitoba R3J 3T2
(*Orders*: Tel: 204 837-2987)

Australia
Blackwell Science Pty Ltd
54 University Street
Carlton, Victoria 3053
(*Orders*: Tel: 3 9347 0300
           Fax: 3 9347 5001)

A catalogue record for this title
is available from the British Library

ISBN 0-632-05044-6

Library of Congress
Cataloging in Publication Data

Data interpretation questions in
pediatrics/Fiona Finlay ... [et al.]
          p.   cm.
   Includes bibliographical references.
   ISBN 0-632-05044-6. — ISBN
   0632-05044-6
   1. Pediatrics — Examinations,
questions, etc.
   2. Children — Diseases —
Diagnosis — Examinations, questions,
etc.
   I. Finlay, Fiona, MRCP.
   [DNLM: 1. Diagnosis,
   Differential —
   in infancy & childhood.
   2. Pediatrics case studies.
   3. Pediatrics examination
   questions.
   WS 141 D232 1998]
   RJ48.2.D37   1998
   618.92′00076 — dc21
   DNLM/DLC
   for Library of Congress   98-21391
                                       CIP

CONTENTS

PREFACE

Data interpretation is part of daily paediatric practice. Questions on data interpretation form one part of paediatric postgraduate examinations. We hope this book will help those preparing for these examinations and that it will stimulate further thought and discussion.

We have tried to include questions on a wide range of common exam topics followed by answers—a short discussion section and references to encourage further reading. Some questions are straightforward and others are more complex.

The answers we have given are those which we feel are most appropriate for the history and data given, although there may be other answers which could be considered correct.

Good Luck!

FF, LL, SL, JC

The standard texts referred to throughout the book are:
Forfar & Arneil's Textbook of Paediatrics (eds A.G.M. Campbell and N. McIntosh), 4th edn, 1992. Churchill Livingstone.
Nelson's Textbook of Paediatrics (eds W.E. Nelson, R.E. Behrman, R.M. Kliegman and A.M. Arvin), 15th edn, 1996. W.B. Saunders.
Roberton's Textbook of Neonatology (ed. N.R.C. Roberton), 2nd edn, 1992. Churchill Livingstone.

PREFACE

Data interpretation is part of daily paediatric practice. Questions on data interpretation form one part of paediatric postgraduate examinations. We hope this book will help those preparing for these examinations and that it will stimulate further thought and discussion.

We have tried to include questions on a wide range of common exam topics followed by answers—a short discussion section and references to encourage further reading. Some questions are straightforward and others are more complex.

The answers we have given are those which we feel are most appropriate for the history and data given, although there may be other answers which could be considered correct.

Good Luck!

FF, LL, SL, JC

The standard texts referred to throughout the book are:
Forfar & Arneil's Textbook of Paediatrics (eds A.G.M. Campbell and N. McIntosh), 4th edn, 1992. Churchill Livingstone.
Nelson's Textbook of Paediatrics (eds W.E. Nelson, R.E. Behrman, R.M. Kliegman and A.M. Arvin), 15th edn, 1996. W.B. Saunders.
Roberton's Textbook of Neonatology (ed. N.R.C. Roberton), 2nd edn, 1992. Churchill Livingstone.

QUESTIONS

A 4-year-old girl arrived in casualty unconscious, accompanied by her grandmother. She had been pyrexial all day and on arrival her temperature was 38.5°C and her respiratory rate was 50/min.

Investigations showed:

Serum sodium	144 mmol/l
Serum bicarbonate	9 mmol/l
Serum glucose	4.1 mmol/l
CSF lymphocytes	3×10^6/l
CSF protein	0.5 g/l
CSF glucose	3.6 mmol/l

a What is the most likely diagnosis?
b Name two relevant investigations.
c What treatment is required?

A 14-month-old girl was referred to outpatients with a poor appetite and general lethargy. She had been breast fed until the age of 4 months when solids were introduced. Initially she was keen to try new foods but as the variety of foods offered broadened, she became disinterested in eating. On examination she was a pretty fair-haired girl on the 3rd centile for weight and 50th centile for height. Her abdomen was soft with no organomegaly but was rather protuberant.

Investigations are as follows:

Haemoglobin	9.5 g/dl
White blood count	9.2×10^9/l
Platelets	294×10^9/l
Film	microcytic, hypochromic
Free T4	22 pmol/l
TSH	3.9 µmol/l

Anti-gliadin antibodies   present
Antiendomesial antibodies   present

a What is the likely diagnosis?
b What test would confirm your diagnosis?
c Suggest two causes for the anaemia.

---

3 A 14-year-old boy is admitted with a diagnosis of a right lower lobe pneumonia. After 2 days of intravenous penicillin he is less pyrexial but his heart rate and respiratory rate are rising.

The following lung function test results are obtained:

	Actual (l)	Predicted (l)
FVC	1.1	2.4
FEV1	1.03	2.21
FEV1/FVC (%)	93.6	

a What type of respiratory impairment does this show?
b What complication has arisen?
c Name three other conditions which would give similar lung function test results.

---

4 A 15-year-old girl has had poor school performance recently and difficult behaviour. She presents to the school nurse with malaise, weight loss and mildly yellow sclera. On examination her liver can be palpated 3 cm below the costal margin, and she is noted to be clumsy with an intention tremor.

Investigations:

Bilirubin	275 µmol/l
Aspartate aminotransferase	217 IU/l
Prothrombin time	9 s (<4 s)

Urinary glucose ++

a What is the likely diagnosis?
b What further pathognomonic sign may be found on examination?
c What further diagnostic tests may be performed?

You are asked to assess an 11-year-old boy who has not made as much progress as expected during his years at junior school. He has good general health with no sensory problems and his parents are of normal intelligence.

He can:

- accurately draw a square and a triangle, but not a diamond;
- count backwards from 10 but not 20;
- tell the time to the nearest hour only;
- distinguish 'long' and 'short' but not 'heavy' and 'light'.

a What is his developmental age?
b What signs would you look for on physical examination?
c What is the most likely diagnosis?

A 3-year-old boy is referred to a paediatrician following his 3 year assessment as his mother is concerned that he is clumsy. On examination he looks well but is noted to fall frequently and to be toe walking.

Investigations are as follows:

Haemoglobin	13.2 g/dl
White blood count	5.6×10^9/l
Platelets	334×10^9/l
CPK	13 405 IU/l

a What is the most probable diagnosis?
b What specific sign would you look for?
c What further investigations would you arrange?

7 A 3-day-old baby boy was born with no complications and bottle fed well for the first 2 days. On day 3 he became irritable, refused feeds and started vomiting. On examination he was drowsy, tachypnoeic and having momentary seizures. One male sibling had died at the age of 2 days — cause unknown.

Blood results:

ammonia	254 µM (< 35 µM)
pH	7.35
liver function tests	normal parameters
septic screen	negative

a Give two investigations to aid diagnosis.
b What is the most likely diagnosis?
c How would you manage this baby?

8 A 2-year-old boy presented to casualty with a chest infection. On examination he was noted to have widespread eczema and scattered bruises.

Investigations:

Haemoglobin	8.8 g/dl
White blood count	8.8×10^9/l
Platelets	67×10^9/l
IgG levels	normal
IgM levels	reduced
IgA levels	elevated
IgE levels	elevated

a What is the diagnosis?
b What is the inheritance pattern?
c Why is he anaemic?

A 7-year-old girl with no significant past medical history has an ECG performed following unexplained fainting episodes at home and at school.

a What abnormalities are illustrated in the ECG shown in Fig. 1?
b What condition does she have?
c What further investigation may be performed?

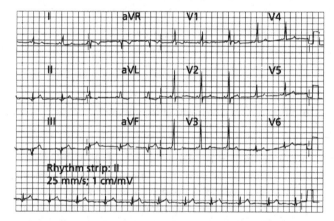

Fig. 1

Two unrelated children are referred to the genetics clinic. Sarah is 3 years old and has marked developmental delay and epilepsy. On examination she has microcephaly and ataxia.

Nathan is 8 months old. In the neonatal period he was very floppy and he is now failing to thrive.

Both children had blood samples sent for chromosomal analysis and the results are as follows:

• deletion in the q 11–13 region of chromosome 15.

a What condition does Sarah have?
b What condition does Nathan have?

---

11 A general practitioner refers a 12-year-old girl with a persistent vaginal discharge that is resistant to treatment with amoxicillin and local steroid preparations. On examination the girl has breast buds and a little pubic hair and her perineum looks normal.

There is a moderate amount of vaginal discharge—non-offensive and green-yellow with the following characteristics:

pH	4.0
epithelial cells	occasional
white cells	occasional
Gram-positive cocci	+++

a How would you treat this child?
b What further investigation is indicated?

---

12 A 5-year-old boy is referred to a cardiology clinic as a heart murmur is detected at a routine school entry medical. He has been well in the past with no significant medical history. On clinical examination in outpatients his heart rate is 90 beats/min and blood pressure 90/60. There is a systolic murmur which is loudest in the pulmonary area and there is a widely split second sound.

Investigations reveal:

Chest X-ray	large heart pulmonary plethora
ECG	RSR′ pattern in the chest leads right axis

a What is the diagnosis?
b What treatment is required?

A 12-year-old boy with cystic fibrosis regularly had **13** *Pseudomonas aeruginosa* cultured from his sputum. This has always been successfully treated with physiotherapy and antibiotics. He now presents with a 5-day history of shortness of breath, wheeze, fever and an irritant cough.

a Name two important investigations.
b What is the most likely diagnosis?

A 19-month-old infant presents with severe seborrhoeic **14** dermatitis on his scalp and chest. Examination reveals enlarged nodes in the axilla and groin, with a moderately enlarged liver and spleen. His general health is good, with no admissions to hospital. He attended the accident and emergency department on one occasion following a fall from a slide and a skull X-ray showed a lytic lesion but no skull fractures.

Investigations reveal:

Haemoglobin	11.5 g/dl
White blood count	7.7×10^9/l
Platelets	245×10^9/l

a What is the diagnosis?
b What further investigations are required?
c What is the treatment?

A 7-year-old boy is referred to the immunization clinic. He **15** has previously lived in Bhutan and his family are about to return to live there. His parents want to know if he should have a BCG vaccine before they travel. He has a Heaf test and the results are read 72 hours later.

The result shows that the centre of the reaction is filled with induration, forming a disc 7 mm wide.

a In the light of this result should the BCG vaccination be given?
b Are there any other vaccines which he should have other than the routine childhood vaccines?

16 A 7-year-old girl was admitted with gross haematuria. All her family had suffered sore throats over the past few days.

Tests revealed:

Urea	3.9 mmol/l
Sodium	135 mmol/l
Potassium	4.0 mmol/l
Urine microscopy	red cell casts ++
	granular casts ++
Creatinine clearance	92 ml/min
Urinary protein	0.18 g/24 h

a Suggest two useful investigations.
b What is the most likely diagnosis?

17 A baby is admitted to the neonatal unit from the ward with poor feeding, bilateral talipes and generalized hypotonia. The delivery was normal, birth weight 3.4 kg, but polyhydramnios had been noted in pregnancy. Both parents are well but mother has mild learning difficulties. Their first child died at the age of 14 weeks following a respiratory infection.

Investigations were as follows:

Full septic screen   normal

Haemoglobin	18.2 g/dl
White blood count	6.4 × 10⁹/l
Platelets	287 × 10⁹/l
Sodium	139 mmol/l
Potassium	4.1 mmol/l
Corrected calcium	2.35 mmol/l

a What is the most likely diagnosis?
b Name three investigations which may be helpful.

a Describe the karyotype shown in Fig. 2.
b Describe three phenotypical features of this condition.
c What further investigations would you perform?

18

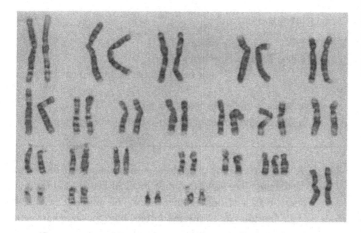

Fig. 2

A sweat test was carried out on a 3-year-old girl with a chronic cough who was failing to gain weight and slow to meet her developmental milestones.

19

Sweat test results:

Weight of sweat   75 mg

Sodium	105 mmol/l
Chloride	60 mmol/l
Potassium	13 mmol/l

a How would you interpret these results?
b Suggest the next useful investigation.

20 A 14-year-old boy attends his general practitioner with a chest infection. On auscultation of the chest there is an ejection systolic click which is loudest at the left sternal border. There is a thrill parasternally and in the suprasternal notch. His heart rate is 80 beats/min and blood pressure 90/65 mmHg.

Investigations:

ECG	normal
Chest X-ray	normal size
	left heart border rounded near the apex

a What is the most likely diagnosis?
b What advice would you give to this young man?

21 A 12-year-old boy presented with malaise and recurrent headaches. There was no past medical history of note but there was a strong family history of migraine. General examination was unremarkable but the paediatrician thought he was slightly jaundiced and therefore arranged liver function tests, which gave the following results:

- Bilirubin 70 µmol/l (90% unconjugated)
- ALT 25 IU/l
- Alk phos 310 IU/l
- Albumin 39 g/l
- Total protein 60 g/l

a What is the most likely diagnosis?
b How would you treat this?

---

a Describe the EEG shown in Fig. 3.   **22**
b What is the diagnosis?

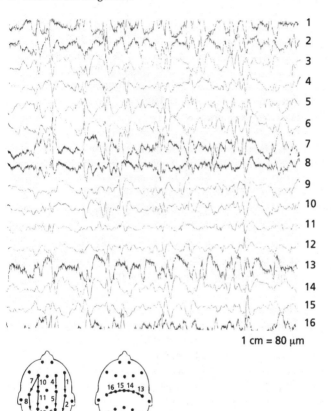

1 cm = 80 μm

Fig. 3

A 16-year-old girl has a 10-day history of fever accompanied   **23**
by tiredness, anorexia, headache and more latterly a sore

throat. On examination she has pharyngitis, generalized lymphadenopathy and a palpable spleen tip.

Investigations reveal:

Haemoglobin	9.9 g/dl
White blood count	19.2×10^9/l (20% neutrophils, 34% lymphocytes, 10% monocytes, 3% eosinophils, 33% atypical mononuclear cells)
Platelets	120×10^9/l
Reticulocyte count	6%

a What is the probable diagnosis?
b What tests should be done to confirm this?

24 A term neonate weighing 3.4 kg has Apgar scores of 2 at 1 min, 2 at 3 min, 6 at 5 min and 9 at 10 min. He is admitted to the neonatal unit where he is given intravenous fluids as he is a poor feeder. Over the first 48 h he shows little improvement and investigations show:

Plasma:
Sodium	107 mmol/l
Potassium	3.4 mmol/l
Urea	1.2 mmol/l
Calcium	1.76 mmol/l
Phosphate	1.28 mmol/l
Protein	50 g/l
Albumin	25 g/l
Bilirubin	92 µmol/l
Alk phos	237 IU/l

Urine:
Sodium	3 mmol/l
Potassium	33 mmol/l

| Urea | 73 mmol/l |
| Osmolality | 450 mosmol/kg |

a What is the diagnosis?
b What is the most likely cause?
c What treatment is required?

Study the family tree shown in Fig. 4.

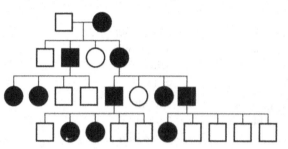

Fig. 4

a What is the inheritance?
b Name one condition which illustrates this inheritance pattern?

A routine filter paper blood spot TSH was elevated in an 8-day-old baby born at term weighing 3.35 kg.

Further serum analysis revealed:

• free T4 <1 pmol/l (normal range 8–26 pmol/l)
• free T3 1.3 pmol/l (normal range 3–9 pmol/l)

Analysis of maternal TSH, T4 and T3 were all within the normal range.

a What is the diagnosis?
b What treatment is necessary?

A 2-year-old boy is referred to social services by his day nursery, with a black eye. His parents are adamant that the bruising occurred spontaneously and that he has not been injured in any way, either accidentally or non-accidentally. They also report that he has been irritable and lethargic over the past weeks. On examination he has periorbital bruising and an abdominal mass is palpable.

Investigations reveal:

Sodium	139 mmol/l
Potassium	3.4 mmol/l
Urea	3.1 mmol/l
Creatinine	37 µmol/l
Haemoglobin	7.6 g/dl
White blood count	7.9×10^9/l
Platelets	176×10^9/l

a What is the most likely diagnosis?
b What tests would help you confirm this?

An infant has a normal delivery but has difficulty establishing feeds. On day 4 she appears very sleepy and is admitted to the neonatal unit following a prolonged apnoea.

Initial investigations show:

Plasma:

Sodium	143 mmol/l
Potassium	4.1 mmol/l
Urea	1.8 mmol/l
Creatinine	39 µmol/l
Alk phos	364 IU/l
ALT	31 IU/l
Glucose	3.7 mmol/l

QUESTIONS

CRP	2.1 µmol/l
Glycine	745 µmol/l (< 575 µmol/l)

Urine:
Culture	no growth
Glucose	negative
Ketones	negative

Further investigations reveal:
Plasma glycine	745 µmol/l (< 575 µmol/l)
CSF glycine	155 µmol/l (< 13 mmol/)

a What is the diagnosis?
b What is the prognosis for this infant?

A mother requests a school entry medical as her 5-year-old daughter is complaining of tiredness and she has a very poor appetite. On examination she was noted to be slightly jaundiced with an enlarged spleen.

Investigations reveal:

Haemoglobin	7.3 g/dl
White blood count	8.2×10^9/l
Platelets	419×10^9/l
Reticulocytes	12%
Total bilirubin	71 µmol/l

Direct Coombs test	negative
Red cell osmotic fragility	shift of curve to the right

a What is the most probable diagnosis?
b What is the inheritance?
c What treatment is required?

A 12-year-old boy attends his local casualty department with abdominal/back pain. He is diagnosed as suffering from renal colic and an X-ray reveals nephrocalcinosis.

His height is on the 3rd centile and his weight on the 25th centile. General examination is unremarkable.
Blood results are as follows:

Sodium	139 mmol/l
Potassium	2.6 mmol/l
Urea	5.8 mmol/l
Creatinine	122 µmol/l
Glucose	5.3 mmol/l
Chloride	124 mmol/l
Arterial pH	7.21

a What is the most likely diagnosis?
b What other investigations would you perform?

---

31 A 6-week-old baby girl is admitted for investigation of recurrent seizures. She is found to have hepatomegaly but no other clinical abnormalities.

Serum results are as follows:

Bicarbonate	14 mmol/l
Glucose	1.8 mmol/l
Triglycerides	6.6 mmol/l (0.6–1.7 mmol/l)
Cholesterol	16.2 mmol/l (2.4–5.6 mmol/l)

a What is the most likely diagnosis?
b How is the diagnosis made?
c What is the prognosis?

---

32 A 15-year-old boy who is a keen bodybuilder attends his general practitioner complaining of feeling nauseous and generally 'off form', with loss of appetite. He denies the use of anabolic steroids but he is usually on a high protein diet with vitamin supplementation. He looks pale but examination is otherwise unremarkable.

The following results are obtained on investigation:

Haemoglobin	9.4 g/dl
Corrected calcium	2.92 mmol/l
Creatinine	188 µmol/l

a What is the most likely diagnosis?
b What other investigations are required?

A 14-year-old boy has a long history of increasing fatigue. **33**
Clinically he is found to have a murmur. Cardiac catheter
data is as outlined below.

Site	Oxygen saturation (%)	Pressure (mmHg)
SVC	55	
RA	60	8 mean
IVC	65	
RV	60	90
PA	60	85/50 mean 62
LA		20 mean
LV	98	120/8
Aorta	98	120/80

a What cardiac lesion is illustrated by the catheter data?
b In what position will the murmur be heard best?

A 38-week gestation breast-fed infant weighing 3.3 kg is **34**
noted to be jaundiced at 74 h of age.

The investigations are as follows:

Total bilirubin	154 µmol/l
Haemoglobin	19.7 g/dl
White blood count	17.3×10^9/l
Platelets	227×10^9/l
Direct Coombs test	negative
Urine microscopy	normal

Urine clinitest   negative

a What treatment is required?
b What is the most likely diagnosis?

---

35 A 9-year-old boy with long standing lung disease had lung function tests carried out:

	Pre-salbutamol	Post-salbutamol	Predicted
FVC (l)	2.0	2.1	2.4
FEV1 (l)	1.2	1.6	2.0
RV (l)	1.3	1.0	0.6
TLC (l)	3.3	3.2	3.0

a What are the three physiological abnormalities illustrated here?
b Name two laboratory techniques used to measure total lung volumes.

---

36 A 5-year-old girl is referred to the growth clinic with short stature. A blood sample is sent to the cytogenetics laboratory.

The report reads as follows:

Karyotype 45X/46XX

a What diagnosis is suggested by this report?
b What clinical features would you look for?
c What other investigations would you arrange?

---

37 A 17-year-old was referred by his general practitioner with prominent nipples. He was being bullied at school and had recently started weight training to develop a more 'macho' image. He had been seen by the school doctor one year previously and reassured that the problem would go away but instead his breasts had got larger. The general

practitioner had done some initial investigations as he was
unsure to whom to refer.

FSH   7 IU/l (1–11 IU/l)
LH   4 IU/l (1–7 IU/l)
Testosterone   15 nmol/l (10–30 nmol/l)
Oestradiol   54 pmol/l (37–129 pmol/l)

On examination his height and weight are on the 50th centile
and he has stage 5 pubic hair development. His testicular
volume is 6 ml and breast tissue is 3.5 cm bilaterally.

a What is the diagnosis?
b What causes need to be considered?
c How should this condition be managed?

A new inflammatory mediator is discovered and pro-
visionally called 'rheublam'. In order to assess its ability
to discriminate between children with disease and those
without, a sample of normal healthy boys (aged 5–15
years) is randomly chosen from the whole population of
the same age and sex.

Results are normally distributed and show a mean value
of 'rheublam' to be 16.4 g/dl with a standard deviation of
4.2 g/dl.

A single-handed general practitioner with a practice list
of 2000 has 500 boys age 5–15 on his list.

a How many would you expect to have a serum
'rheublam' greater than 24.8 g/dl and less than 12.2 g/dl?
b How big would this general practitioner's list of 5–15-
year-old boys have to be before he would expect to see an
individual with a value greater than 29.0 g/dl?
c What percentage will have a value of 20.6 g/dl or
less?

A 1-year-old boy with tetralogy of Fallot undergoes a   **39** routine general anaesthetic for removal of his adenoids. As he is being induced he becomes severely cyanosed, bradycardiac and hypotensive (60/25). His arterial gases indicate a marked metabolic acidosis.

a What caused his marked deterioration?
b How would you manage this situation?

40 An 8-month-old girl presents with an 8-day history of fever, rash, cervical adenitis and pharyngitis.

The following results were obtained:

- throat swab — beta haemolytic *Streptococcus* not isolated
- full blood count — haemoglobin 11.2 g/dl
  white blood count 18.6×10^9/l
  platelets 1157×10^9/l

a What diagnosis should be considered?
b What critical complications may arise?
c What treatment may be given?

41 A 3-year-old girl who is recovering from chickenpox develops a headache, becomes confused and starts vomiting.

The following results are obtained on investigation:

Urea	4.9 mmol/l
Sodium	131 mmol/l
Potassium	4.4 mmol/l
Bicarbonate	29 mmol/l
Blood sugar	1.2 mmol/l
ALT	126 IU/l (7–55 IU/l)
Ammonia	512 µmol/l
PTT	elevated

a What further investigation would confirm the diagnosis?
b What is the diagnosis?

A 15-year-old boy presents with poor concentration at **42** school and increasing frontal headaches for 3 weeks. His parents separated 2 months ago and he is living with his father who is a cattleman.

On physical examination he has acne on his face and back. He has no neurological signs on gross or fine motor testing, reflexes and sensory and motor functions are normal but bilateral papilloedema is present. His blood pressure is normal.

Investigations reveal:

Haemoglobin	12.3 g/dl
White blood count	$8.7 \times 10^9/l$
Platelets	$244 \times 10^9/l$
Sodium	143 mmol/l
Potassium	4.1 mmol/l
Urea	3.3 mmol/l
Calcium	2.43 mmol/l
Bilirubin	11 μmol/l
ALP	35 IU/L

a What other clinical examination should be performed?
b What important history is missing?
c What is the likely diagnosis?
d How should he be treated?

A 9-month-old Turkish boy is admitted with jaundice, **43** pallor and failure to thrive. He is found to have hepato-splenomegaly.

Results show:

Haemoglobin   3.7 g/dl

23

White blood count	7.7×10^9/l
Platelets	210×10^9/l
Reticulocytes	8%
Total bilirubin	103 µmol/L
Direct bilirubin	17 µmol/l
Bone marrow	Erythroid hyperplasia, dyserythropoiesis, red cell inclusions
Blood film	Microcytosis, poikilocytosis, target cells, nucleated red cells +++
Electrophoresis	Hb F 90%
	Hb A2 5%
	Hb A absent

a What is the diagnosis?
b What treatment is required?
c Name four potential complications which should be considered during follow up?

---

44 A 15-year-old male presents with a 3-week history of frequency and dysuria. On examination he is 70 kg, 163 cm tall and his blood pressure is 130/75.

His urine sample on testing is:

Nitrite screen	negative
White blood cells	+++
Gram stain	negative

a What are the likely causes of his dysuria?
b What else should you ask him?
c Are any further investigations required?
d What treatment is needed?

---

45 A 2-month-old girl presents at the accident and emergency department with a 2-day history of vomiting and laboured breathing. On examination she is underweight and looks pale, shocked and lethargic. She is apyrexial with a heart rate of 147/min and a respiratory rate of 50/min.

Arterial blood gas results are as follows:

pH	7.06
pO_2	12.3 kPa
pCO_2	2.9 kPa
Bicarbonate	7 mmol/l
Chest X-ray	normal
Cardio-thoracic ratio	50%

a What is the likely diagnosis?
b What initial treatment is required?
c What further investigations are required?

---

46 A 33-week gestation baby girl is born following spontaneous onset of labour. She does not require resuscitation immediately but later on SCBU needs CPAP. On day 8 she develops tachypnoea and a loud long systolic murmur is heard all over the precordium. Her liver is palpated 4 cm below the costal margin.

a What is the likely diagnosis?
b Outline your management.
c What are the possible side-effects of the main drug used?

---

47 In a developing country there is an outbreak of cholera affecting adults and children. There are 4000 births in 1 year. Six hundred of these are stillbirths, 400 die in the first week, 200 die between the first and fourth weeks and a further 600 die between the first month and the first year.

a What is the infant mortality rate?
b What is the neonatal mortality rate?
c What is the perinatal mortality rate?

---

48 An 8-year-old boy is hit by a van while cycling and sustains head and chest injuries. He is resuscitated and ventilated and at 24 h post-injury is in a stable condition with good arterial blood gases.

Thirty-six hours post-injury he starts to develop a tachycardia and his central venous pressure and blood pressure start to fall.

Investigations at this time are as follows:

Haemoglobin	15.5 g/dl
White blood count	12.3×10^9/l
Platelets	150×10^9/l
Sodium	150 mmol/l
Potassium	5.6 mmol/l
Chloride	123 mmol/l
Bicarbonate	17 mmol/l
Urinary osmolality	55 mosm/kg

a What is the diagnosis?
b What treatment is required?

---

49 Look at the pedigree outlined below in Fig. 5.

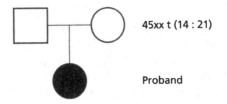

45xx t (14 : 21)

Proband

Fig. 5

a What is the likely karyotype of this proband?
b What is the syndrome?

A clinically well 4-year-old girl is referred with a murmur. **50**
Cardiac catheterization data are as outlined below.

Site	Sat (%)	Pressure (mmHg)
RA	70	4 mean
RV	72	23
PA	72	25/10 mean 13
LA	—	8 mean
LV	98	210/10
Asc aorta	97	125/95
Dsc aorta	98	85/50

a What is the diagnosis?

A 20-month-old boy who has one sister presents with **51**
recurrent skin infections and generalized lymphadenopathy. On examination he is found to have moderate
hepatosplenomegaly.

Investigations are as follows:

Haemoglobin	9.1 g/dl		
White blood count	14.4×10^9/l		
Differential		Neutrophils	10.8×10^9/l
		Monocytes	2.1×10^9/l
		Lymphocytes	1.5×10^9/l
Platelets	205×10^9/l		
MCV	84 fl		
Film	Neutrophil leucocytosis with toxic granulation of neutrophils		
Immunoglobulins	All raised		

Nitro-blue tetrazolium test (NBT) — reduced rate of formation of purple formazen

a What is the most likely diagnosis?
b Which members of the family might also have an abnormal NBT test?

52   **a** How old are the brothers who drew the men shown in Fig. 6.

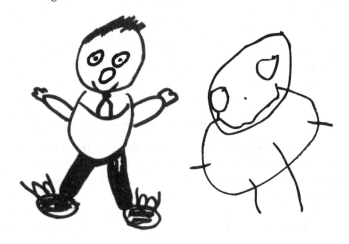

Fig. 6

53   A 2-week-old Spanish girl is brought to the ward sweating and vomiting. She was born to unrelated parents and breast fed extremely well until the day of admission. Twelve hours previously she had been well but posseting and her parents had given her diluted fruit juice. On examination she was noted to be tachypnoeic and drowsy with a liver edge 4 cm below the costal margin.

Blood results revealed:

Glucose   1.0 mmol/l

pH   7.14
HCO₃   8 mmol/l

a What is the most likely diagnosis?
b What is its inheritance?
c What would you advise the parents?

A 5-month-old baby attends for follow up with a giant **54** cavernous haemangioma affecting his left shoulder and neck. He is noted to be pale and have a widespread petechial rash.

Initial investigations showed:

Haemoglobin	7.4 g/dl
White blood count	11.2×10^9/l
Platelets	19×10^9/l
Film	Fragmented red cells
INR	1.2
APTT	elevated
Fibrinogen	0.9 g/l
FDPs	raised

a What is the diagnosis?

An 8-year-old soap opera addict spends more time day- **55** dreaming than paying attention in class.

a What is illustrated in her EEG shown in Fig. 7?
b How could you precipitate this if the trace was initially normal?
c What is the treatment of choice?

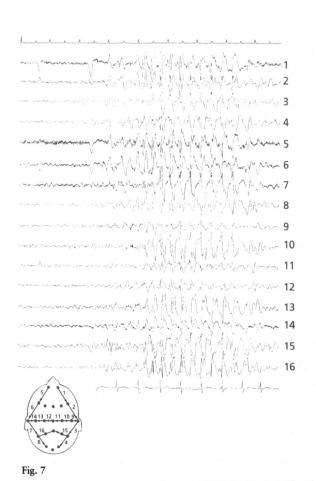

Fig. 7

56 A 6-year-old boy presents with a 1-week history of profuse watery diarrhoea and increasing oedema. Examination confirms widespread oedema, pallor and lethargy. His blood pressure is 147/96, heart rate 101/min and respiratory rate 40/min.

Results are as follows:

Sodium   121 mmol/l

Potassium	8.7 mmol/l
Creatinine	175 µmol/l
Bicarbonate	10 mmol/l
Haemoglobin	6.6 g/dl
White blood count	11.1×10^9/l
Platelets	70×10^9/l
Urine	red blood cells +++
	white cell count +

a What is the likely diagnosis?
b What emergency treatment is needed?
c What short-term treatment may he need?

A 2-year-old Asian child is brought to clinic with poor weight gain and non-specific malaise. He was breast fed until 8 months and then weaned onto ordinary cows' milk. He drinks about 3 pints of milk a day and shows little interest in a solid diet except for crisps and sweets.

Investigations reveal:

Haemoglobin	6.4 g/dl
White blood count	9.7×10^9/l
Platelets	268×10^9/l
MCV	61 fl
Film	microcytic, hypochromic
Ferritin	7 µg/l

a What is the likely diagnosis?
b What condition does the ferritin help distinguish this from?
c What other condition is the child at risk of developing?

A 6-month-old boy was profoundly cyanosed. His cardiac catheterization data are illustrated below.

Site	Oxygen sat (%)	Pressure (mmHg)
SVC	60	
RA	79	4
IVC	61	
RV	80	92
PA	92	20/10
LA	93	4
LV	93	28
Aorta	80	90/60

a What is the abnormality?

---

59 A 3.6 kg baby is noted to be jaundiced at 18 h of age.

Investigations show:

Total bilirubin	148 µmol/l
Haemoglobin	14.8 g/dl
White blood count	22.4×10^9/l
Platelets	370×10^9/l
Infant blood group	A positive
Maternal blood group	O positive
Direct Coombs test (DCT)	negative
Urine	clinitest negative
	microscopy negative

a What is the most likely diagnosis?
b What treatment is required?

---

60 An 11-year-old boy (height 142 cm and weight 75 kg) was investigated following a 4-month history of feeling breathless on exertion. The results of an exercise test with FEV1 measurements are shown.

Time	FEV1
Before	2.91 l
1 min after	3.1 l (predicted value 3.2 l)
5 min after	2.94 l
10 min after	2.90 l
15 min after	3.1 l

a What does this exercise test show?
b What is the most likely explanation for his dyspnoea?

A 13-year-old boy who is performing well in mainstream education is seen in clinic complaining of 'distorted vision'. On examination his weight was on the 50th centile, his height above the 97th centile and his head circumference on the 50th centile. He was noted to have a high arched palate and a heart murmur.

a What is the most likely diagnosis?
b What condition may it be confused with on clinical examination alone?
c What is the cause of his visual problem?
d What is the pathophysiology of the heart murmur?

A 5-week-old girl presents with a cough and recurrent apnoeic spells. A septic screen is performed with results as follows:

Full blood count:

Haemoglobin	12.4 g/dl
White blood count	29.0 × 10^9/l (neutrophils 4.0, lymphocytes 25.0)
Platelets	323 × 10^9/l
CSF	no red cells
	no white cells
	no growth

Blood culture	no growth
Urine culture	no growth
X-ray	streaky appearance of the lung fields

a What diagnosis should be considered?
b What further investigations should be performed?
c How long would this child be infectious for?

---

63 A 3-year-old girl who is usually well presents with pallor and tiredness. On examination there are no significant findings apart from pale mucous membranes.

Initial investigations show:

Haemoglobin	4.1 g/dl		
MCV	86.3 fl		
Reticulocytes	0.2%		
White blood count	$9.3 \times 10^9/l$	Neutrophils	50%
Platelets	$410 \times 10^9/l$		

a What is the most likely diagnosis?
b What further investigations are required?
c What is the likely outcome?

---

64 On examination a 'normal' baby is found to have the following reflex pattern:

Asymmetric tonic neck reflex	absent
Moro reflex	absent
Walking reflex	absent
Grasp reflex	absent
Parachute reflex	absent

a How old is the baby?

A baby born by LSCS at 31 weeks gestation is noted to **65** have grunting respirations at 2 h of age. An arterial blood gas sample revealed the following results:

pH   7.18
pCO_2 9.36 kPa
pO_2 4.33 kPa
BE   −3.9

a What does this blood gas show?
b What is the most likely explanation?
c Name three other conditions which should be considered.

A 16-month-old boy is referred to clinic with a history of **66** intermittent jaundice. Examination reveals an abdominal mass in the right upper quadrant. There is no family history of note. The total bilirubin is 172 μmol/l (conjugated 152 μmol/l).

a What is the most likely diagnosis?
b What further investigation is required?
c What treatment is required?

A boy who initially presented to casualty with abdominal **67** pain was subsequently found to have renal calculi. Analysis of his urine sample by chromatography showed excess lysine, cystine, ornithine and arginine.

a What is the likely diagnosis?
b What clinical complications may arise?
c What treatment is required?

A baby is admitted from the postnatal ward with wide- **68** spread petechial haemorrhages and is subsequently found to have bilateral intraventricular haemorrhages with some dilatation of the ventricles.

Investigations are as follows:

Baby's blood	Haemoglobin	11.2 g/dl
	Platelets	17×10^9/l
	White blood count	19.4×10^9/l
	PLA1	positive
	Blood culture	no growth after 48 h
	TORCH screen	negative
Baby's urine	Microscopy and culture	< 10 white cells
		no red cells
		no organisms
		no growth
Maternal results	Haemoglobin	11.4 g/dl
	Platelets	356×10^9/l
	White blood count	8.3×10^9/l
	PLA1	negative

a What is the diagnosis?
b What treatment is required?

---

69 A ferric chloride test is performed on urine samples from two different children. In the first case the urine turns green, in the second case it turns purple. Give two possible explanations for the colour changes in each case.

---

70 A baby is noted to have mild dysmorphic features and examination reveals an ejection systolic murmur.

Biochemistry revealed:

Sodium	142 mmol/l
Potassium	3.4 mmol/l
Calcium	2.98 mmol/l
Phosphate	1.73 mmol/l
Alkaline phosphate	115 IU/l

a What is the most likely diagnosis?
b What are the two most likely underlying cardiac pathologies?

A 3-year-old boy presented with persistent fever and clinically a left lower lobe pneumonia was detected. He was treated with intravenous penicillin and he improved slowly but relapsed when antibiotics were stopped. He eventually recovered and was discharged only to be admitted 3 months later again with pneumonia.

Investigations on that occasion revealed:

Haemoglobin	10.7 g/dl
White blood count	8.6 × 10⁹/l (neutrophils 36%, lymphocytes 58%, monocytes 5%)
ESR	9
Sweat test	normal
Serum IgG	1.2 U/ml (63–160)
Serum IgA	1.0 U/ml (25–117)
Serum IgM	5.2 U/ml (150–650)
Cell-mediated immunity	normal
Lymphocyte markers	normal T cells, absent B cells

When his younger brother was born he developed numerous ear infections in the first 18 months of life and was subsequently investigated.

a What is the diagnosis?
b What treatment is required?

72 A healthy 4-year-old girl has recurrent nosebleeds at playgroup. She also appears to bruise more easily than her friends.

Investigations are as follows:

Haemoglobin	11.5 g/dl
White blood count	8.5 g/dl
Platelets	310×10^9/l
Blood film	normal
Coagulation screen	normal
Bleeding time	19 min

a What is the most likely diagnosis?
b What specific investigation is required to confirm this diagnosis?
c What is the inheritance pattern?

73 A 4-month-old infant was referred with failure to thrive. A murmur was heard on auscultation and therefore cardiac catheterization was performed.

The following results were obtained:

Site	Oxygen saturation (%)	Pressure (mmHg)
RA	75	4 mean
RV	79	85
PA	92	80/25
LA	98	5 mean
LV	95	85
Aorta	92	80/25

a What is the most likely abnormality?
b In which syndrome is this found?

A 3-year-old girl was referred to the child development centre with developmental delay. Her height was on the 50th centile and her weight above the 90th centile. She was noted to have some facial dysmorphic features.

Serum biochemistry revealed:

Calcium	1.21 mmol/l
Phosphate	2.92 mmol/l
Alk phos	292 IU/l
Total protein	63 g/l
Albumin	36 g/l
PTH	normal

There was an absent urinary cAMP response, plasma calcium response and absent urinary phosphate response to a PTH infusion.

a What is the diagnosis?
b What X-rays may be of diagnostic value?
c What would they show?

Laura is noted to have bilateral inguinal swellings at her 6- week check which increase in size when she cries. She is otherwise well with no other abnormalities on examination. She has a 14-year older sister, Amy, who also had inguinal hernias as a baby, and they were repaired at the age of 18 months. Amy has not yet started her periods. Laura also has a 9-year-old brother Alan and a 5-year-old sister Claire.

In view of her unusual problem and a family history of similar problems in her older sister, chromosomal analysis is performed on Laura and her siblings.

Chromosomes	Amy	46XY
	Alan	46XY
	Claire	46XX
	Laura	46XY

a What is the diagnosis?
b What treatment is required?

---

76 In a 2-year cohort study looking at the effect of parental smoking on the incidence of deaths from meningococcal meningitis, the following results were obtained:

	Deaths from meningitis
Smokers (2000)	15
Non-smokers (8000)	30

a What is the risk ratio of smoking?
b What is the odds ratio?
c What is the rate difference?
(**NB** Leave answers as whole fractions)

---

77 Study the family tree shown in Fig. 8.

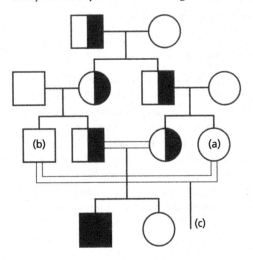

Fig. 8

a What is the inheritance?
b What is the chance of (a) being a carrier?

c What is the chance of (b) being a carrier?
d What is the chance of (c) being affected?

An 11-month-old child of Afro-Carribean parents is **78** admitted with irritability which his parents think is due to abdominal pain. He is found to be pale and mildly icteric with a swollen hand. His abdomen is tender although there is no organomegaly.

Tests revealed the following findings:

Haemoglobin	7.2 g/dl		
MCV	92 fl		
White blood count	$14.7 \times 10^9/l$	Neutrophils	$10.1 \times 10^9/l$
		Lymphocytes	$2.9 \times 10^9/l$
Platelets	$401 \times 10^9/l$		
Reticulocytes	9%		

a What is your provisional diagnosis?
b What would you expect to find on blood film?
c What test would you do to confirm the diagnosis?

A boy is referred to outpatients for investigation. He is **79** generally well but had been complaining of headaches over the previous few months, occurring both during school holidays and term time. Examination revealed pale fundi and mild truncal unsteadiness. Several investigations were performed including an EEG.

a Describe the EEG shown in Fig. 9.
b What conditions would lead to such an EEG pattern?
c What further investigation is required?

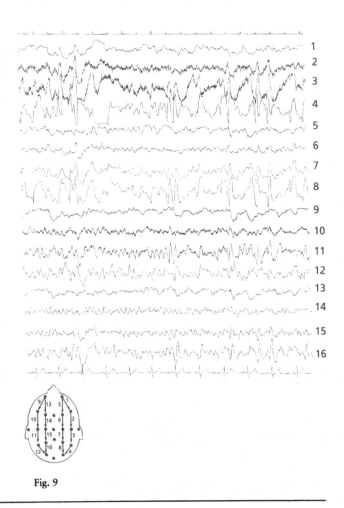

Fig. 9

80 A 4.2 kg infant born at 37 weeks gestation to an insulin-dependent diabetic mother was noticed to have haematuria on nappy changing, at 14 h of age. The baby was slightly tachypnoeic, had normal blood pressure and a palpable abdominal mass.

The following results were obtained on investigation:

Haemoglobin	16.1 g/dl
White blood count	$10.7 \times 10^9/l$
Platelets	$70 \times 10^9/l$
Packed cell volume	78%
Sodium	134 mmol/l
Potassium	5.1 mmol/l
Urea	9.1 mmol/l
Creatinine	187 µmol/l
Glucose	3.4 mmol/l

a What is the likely cause?
b What is the next investigation?
c How would you manage this baby?

---

a What is the technique shown in Fig. 10?
b What is illustrated in this example?
c Name two conditions which illustrate this.

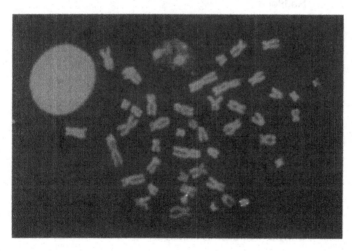

Fig. 10

82 Mary can build a tower of seven bricks and draw in circular scribbles. She knows that she is a girl. However, she cannot draw a circle or make a bridge from bricks.

a What is Mary's developmental age?

83 A 4-year-old girl presents with a 1-month history of swollen eyes. She had been given 'eye drops' by her general practitioner which had not helped to reduce the swelling. On further questioning she said that her throat was 'a bit sore' and her mother said that she had complained over the past few days that her trousers were too tight.

Investigations revealed the following results:

Urine:
Protein   ++++
No blood

Blood:
Sodium   132 mmol/l
Potassium   4.9 mmol/l
Urea   15.8 mmol/l
Albumin   7 g/l
Calcium   2.05 mmol/l
Haemoglobin   13.0 g/dl
White blood count 22.2×10^9/l
Platelets 342×10^9/l

a What is the diagnosis?
b What are the two major complications which may occur?
c What treatment is required?

84 Routine hepatitis screening of a pregnant female reveals the following result:
HBsAg — positive   HBeAg — positive

a What precautions should be taken at birth?
b How should the infant be managed?
c What advice should be given with regard to breast feeding?

A haematology report on a 5-year-old girl admitted with diarrhoea and vomiting is returned to the ward reading 'target cells seen'.   **85**

a What conditions would account for such a report?

A 4-year-old girl presents to your clinic with a 3-month history of constipation. On examination you note that her height is below the 3rd centile, her nipples are widely spaced and there is a 2/6 systolic murmur in the pulmonary area.   **86**

a What are the two most likely diagnoses?
b Give the most common cardiac abnormality in each case.

A 6-year-old boy attended his GP with a 3-month history of lethargy. On examination he looked pale. A blood count was as follows: **87**

Haemoglobin	5.8 g/dl
White blood count	63×10^9/l (neutrophils 14%, lymphocytes 14%, lymphoblasts 71%)
Platelets	110×10^9/l

a What is the most likely diagnosis?
b Give three poor prognostic features of this condition in general.

A 16-year-old adolescent attends casualty having fallen off a tractor on his father's farm. He landed on a rusty nail and has a puncture wound to his left forearm.

His immunization history is as follows:

Primary course DPT and polio	in infancy
Measles immunization	age 18 months
School entry DT and polio	age 4 years
Measles/rubella	age 13 as part of MR campaign

a What three actions should be taken in casualty?

A 6-year-old is reviewed in clinic. Ocular albinism was noted at the 6-week check and since then there has been recurrent bacterial sepsis and ENT problems.

Results are as follows:

Haemoglobin	11.1 g/dl
Platelets	$139 \times 10^9/l$
White blood count	$2.3 \times 10^9/l$ (neutrophils 0.2, lymphocytes 1.8, monocytes 0.3)
MCV	70 fl
PCV	0.33
IgG	14.4 g/l
IgA	2.7 g/l
IgM	1.2 g/l

Neutrophil function 27% : 79% normal control
Bone marrow—abnormal granules in all myeloid cells
Blood film—multiple large granules within the cytoplasm of neutrophils

Karyotype 46XX

a What is the diagnosis?
b Give two complications which may occur

A 3-year-old boy was found to have a murmur by his **90** general practitioner. Cardiac catheterization was carried out and the following results obtained:

Site	Oxygen saturation (%)	Pressure (mmHg)
SVC	70	
RA	85	5 mean
IVC	72	
RV	88	22/10
PA	88	23/11
LA	98	5 mean
LV	97	85
Aorta	97	85/50

a What is the abnormality?
b Name two abnormalities which may be found on a chest X-ray.
c What treatment is required?

A family register with a new general practitioner having **91** lived abroad for the past 3 years. The 6-year-old boy has had the following immunizations:

• Diphtheria, pertussis, tetanus (DPT) and polio age 2 months
• DPT and polio age 4 months
• DPT and polio age 6 months

a Should he have a booster dose of DPT and polio now?
b Should he have the Hib vaccine?
c Should he have any other immunizations?

A breast-fed male infant is being monitored on the postnatal **92** ward where the staff are concerned that he is vomiting and is jaundiced. He is now 5 days old and he had a normal 'first day check' 12 h after delivery.

Investigations are as follows:

Blood:

Sodium	143 mmol/l
Potassium	3.7 mmol/l
Urea	2.8 mmol/l
Creatinine	51 mmol/l
Alk phos	360 IU/l
ALT	172 IU/l
Total bilirubin	380 micromol/l
Conjugated bilirubin	67 micromol/l
Glucose	2.4 mmol/l

Urine:

Multistix	trace of glucose
Clinitest	positive 2%

a What further diagnostic test would you perform?
b What is the most likely diagnosis?
c What treatment is required?

---

93 A 15-year-old girl consults her general practitioner as she wishes to start the oral contraceptive pill. He finds that her blood pressure is 150/95 and on further questioning she admits to frequent headaches, sweating and visual disturbance.

She is referred to outpatients and investigations reveal:

Plasma:

Sodium	141 mmol/l
Potassium	5.9 mmol/l
Urea	4.2 mmol/l

Urine:
24-h metanephrines — elevated

24-h vanillylmandelic acid (VMA)—elevated

a What is the most likely diagnosis?
b What further investigations are required?

A baby has meningitis at the age of 3 weeks and is treated **94** with intravenous antibiotics. He appears to make a full recovery. At follow up in clinic his mother is concerned that he is constantly miserable and despite feeding well, he is not gaining weight.

Investigations show:

Haemoglobin	11.2 g/dl
White blood count	7.4×10^9/l
Platelets	438×10^9/l
CRP	< 0.1

Plasma:

Sodium	158 mmol/l
Potassium	3.7 mmol/l
Urea	5.9 mmol/l
Creatinine	61 µmol/l
Plasma osmolality	355 mosm/l

Urine:

Urine osmolality	127 mosm/l

a What is the probable diagnosis?
b What treatment is required?

Study the pedigree shown in Fig. 11 of a family affected by **95** cystic fibrosis.

If the carrier rate is 1 in 20 what is the chance of

a (a) being a carrier?

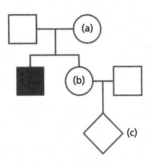

Fig. 11

b (b) being a carrier?
c (c) having cystic fibrosis?

96 A 3.8 kg baby, born by normal vaginal delivery is unexpectedly pale following delivery, although no resuscitation was required. At the age of 1 h he was tachypnoeic and was transferred to the neonatal unit for observation and investigation. On examination the liver edge is 2 cm below the costal margin.

Results:

Haemoglobin	6.1 g/dl
White blood count	$19.2 \times 10^9/l$
Platelets	$227 \times 10^9/l$
Coombs test	negative
Blood film	occasional spherocytes
Kleihauer test	positive
Maternal blood group	O rhesus positive
Baby's blood group	O rhesus positive

Abdominal ultrasound Mild ascites, mildly enlarged liver

a What is the most likely diagnosis?

97 A 4-month-old boy is undergoing investigation for poor weight gain. He was born by normal delivery at term following an uncomplicated pregnancy. On examination cataracts are noted and urine testing gives a positive result with clinitest tablets but a negative result with clinistix.

a Name four substances which if present in the urine would give this result.
b What do clinistix test for?
c What is the most likely diagnosis?

A baby is noted to be jaundiced at his 6-week check. His **98** weight and head circumference are on the 90th centile and there are no concerns about his general development.

Initial investigations reveal:

Total bilirubin	121 µmol/l
Direct bilirubin	100 µmol/l
Alanine aminotransferase	141 IU/l
Aspartate aminotransferase	152 IU/l
Gamma G-T	1005 IU/l
TORCH screen	negative
Hepatitis serology	negative
Urine reducing substances	negative

a What additional information would be valuable in the history and from the examination?
b What would be three investigations of choice?
c What are the differential diagnoses?

You examine a 6-week-old baby girl who has been rushed **99** into hospital. She is tachypnoeic, very poorly perfused and has a heart rate of 310 beats/min. Her liver is palpated 3 cm below the costal margin.

a What is the most likely diagnosis?
b Give three immediate management options.

100 A 12-year-old presents to the emergency clinic with vomiting, dysuria, loin pain and a 10 day history of a flu-like illness, with pyrexia and sore throat. Blood pressure is 130/60.

Investigations reveal:

Urine:
Blood	++
Protein	+
> 20 white cells	
Granular casts	

Blood:
Sodium	139 mmol/l
Potassium	3.7 mmol/l
Urea	31.1 mmol/l
Creatinine	191 μmol/l
Glucose	4.8 mmol/l
Albumin	27 g/l
Protein	60 g/l
Calcium	2.32 mmol/l
Haemoglobin	13.4 g/dl
White blood count	19.9×10^9/l
Platelets	465×10^9/l
CRP	56.6
ASOT	600 IU
C3	0.83 g/dl
C4	0.34 g/dl

a What is the most likely diagnosis?
b What other diagnosis should be considered?
c How would you manage this child?
d What is the prognosis?

101 A 16-year-old boy is concerned that he is not yet entering puberty. He is being teased by friends at school. His father remembers similar peer problems as a youth. On examination he appears a healthy pre-pubescent boy with testicular volume of 4 ml bilaterally.

Examination and investigations:

Height	less than 3rd centile
Weight	3rd centile

Testosterone	0.6 nmol/l (pre-pubertal up to 3.5 nmol/l)
Free T4	21 pmol/l
TSH	2.7 mU/l

Chromosomes	46XY
Bone age	12.9 years
Skull X-ray	normal

a What is the likely diagnosis?
b Would you expect his final adult height to be normal?
c What further investigations are required?

A 19-hour-old, ventilated, 25-week gestation preterm **102** infant, has the following electrolyte values:

Sodium	152 mmol/l
Potassium	3.8 mmol/l
Urea	5.2 mmol/l
Creatinine	71 µmol/l

a What is the most likely cause of this picture?
b What further investigations would you perform?
c How would you manage this baby?

Figure 12 shows the ECG from a 3-year-old boy with a **103** hearing impairment who is being investigated for 'funny turns'.

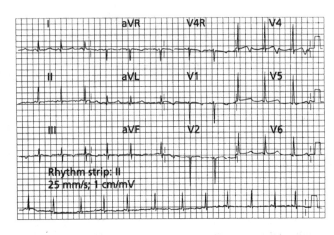

Fig. 12

a What is the main abnormality?
b What syndrome may he have?
c What other syndrome gives a similar ECG?

---

104 The first-born male of non-related parents was found to be profoundly jaundiced on the sixth day of life. He was also vomiting, poorly perfused and hypotonic.

Blood results:

Sodium	118 mmol/l
Potassium	6.0 mmol/l
Chloride	92 mmol/l
Bilirubin	270 mmol/l
Bicarbonate	17 mmol/l
Urea	8.1 mmol/l
Creatinine	92 mmol/l

a What further investigation should be done to confirm the diagnosis?
b What is the diagnosis?
c What treatment is required?

A baby is admitted to the neonatal unit with intrauterine growth retardation and multiple malformations. The karyotype obtained from the baby is shown in Fig. 13.

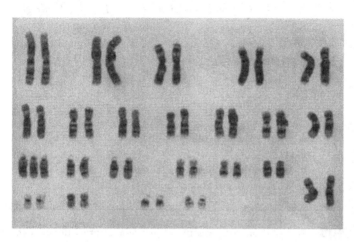

Fig. 13

a Describe this karyotype.
b Describe three phenotypical features of this condition.

At a school medical, a 6-year-old girl is noted to have early breast development and some pubic hair. On questioning her mother says that she has noted blood on her pants several times. General examination is unremarkable apart from several areas of pigmentation on her lower limbs and a small goitre.

Investigations reveal:

TSH   0.1 mU/l (0.3–5.3 mU/l)
T4   251 nmol/l (54–142 nmol/l)

a What syndrome may she have?
b What further investigations would you do to confirm this?

107 An 18-month-old girl attends clinic with a history of shortness of breath and cyanotic spells. Her cardiac catheter data are shown below:

Site	Oxygen saturation (%)	Pressure (mmHg)
RA	60	5 mean
RV	66	85
PA	68	mean 10
LA	98	mean 8
LV	90	85
Aorta	80	85/55

a What structural abnormalities are suggested by these data?
b What is the probable diagnosis?
c What are the treatment options?

108 A 5-year-old girl presents to her general practitioner with a poor appetite and failure to thrive. She is generally well with no significant past medical history. She lives with her parents and two sisters who are also well and there is no family history of note. She has two ponies and the family have three dogs and a cat.

Investigations reveal:

Haemoglobin	8.8 g/dl
Platelets	288×10^9/l
Eosinophils	86×10^9/l
IgM	elevated
IgG	elevated
IgE	elevated

a What is the most likely diagnosis?
b What further investigations are required?
c What treatment is required?

A baby who was born at term following an uncomplicated pregnancy failed his 8-month distraction hearing test and is therefore referred to the hearing clinic. There is no family history of deafness or severe learning difficulties and the child has previously been well. General examination is unremarkable.

a Describe the auditory findings shown in Fig. 14.
b What are the most likely causes?

	Auditory findings	
	Right	Left
High-pitched rattle	No response	No response
'ss'	No response	No response
'bb'/'oo'	55 dBA	60dBA
500 Hz	50	55
1 kHz	60	65
2 kHz	80	85
4 kHz	No response	No response

Fig. 14

110 An 8-year-old boy is brought to hospital by his parents. On checking him before they went to sleep, they found him in bed making grunting sounds, drooling, apparently unable to speak and twitching around the mouth. His EEG is shown in Fig. 15.

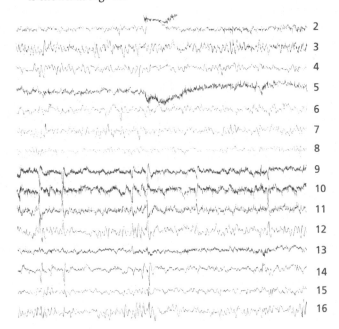

 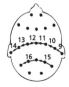

Fig. 15

a What is the diagnosis?
b What is the prognosis?
c What treatment is required?

A 16-year-old girl is investigated for short stature. Clinically she shows no sign of pubertal development.

Anterior pituitary function tests illustrated:

Time (min)	Glucose (mmol/l)	Cortisol (nmol/l)	GH (mU/l)	TSH (mU/l)	LH (U/l)	FSH (U/l)
0	4.6	390	<1	1.8	>25	>50
15	1.8	430	14			
30	0.6	500	20	10.5	>25	>50
45	2.5	620	18			
60	4.0	530	10	7.2	>25	>50

a What is the most likely diagnosis?
b Name one relevant investigation.

An 11-year-old survivor of acute lymphoblastic leukaemia who completed treatment 2 years before presents with increasing breathlessness on exertion. On examination she has a gallop rhythm, a raised respiratory rate and easily palpated liver edge.

Investigations performed showed:

Haemoglobin	12.3 g/dl
White blood count	8.7×10^9/l
Platelets	222×10^9/l
Sodium	134 mmol/l
Potassium	3.6 mmol/l
Urea	5.0 mmol/l
ALP	34 IU/l
ALT	36 IU/l
Bilirubin	9 µmol/l

a What is the likely cause?
b What further investigations are required?

113   A 15-month-old baby is seen in the child development centre. He has a developmental quotient of 60% and progressive hearing loss. Examination is unremarkable apart from marked microcephaly. He was born following an uneventful pregnancy and there is no family history of note.

The results of investigations are as follows:

Chromosomes	balanced translocation
Urine screen	inclusion bodies present

a What is the diagnosis?
b What further investigations are needed?

114   A 32-year-old woman goes into labour during a flu-like illness at 34 weeks' gestation. There was meconium-stained liquor but the baby was born in good condition weighing 2.3 kg with an Apgar score of 8 at 1 min and 9 at 5 min. At 2 h of age he develops respiratory distress.

Investigations reveal:

Chest X-ray	hazy shadowing of both lung fields
Haemoglobin	14.1 g/dl
White cell count	3.5×10^9/l
Platelets	35×10^9/l
Sodium	137 mmol/l
Potassium	4.2 mmol/l
Glucose	5.0 mmol/l
Gastric aspirate	Gram-positive bacillus

a What is the most likely diagnosis?
b What treatment is required?
c What is the prognosis?
d What other information would be useful to obtain from the midwife?

A female infant of Angolan parents presents at the age of 5 weeks with vomiting. Her parents are unrelated and both well and she has a 3-year-old brother who had pyloric stenosis at the age of 6 weeks. She weighed 3.1 kg at birth and she now weighs 5.1 kg and is being fed 190 ml of whey-dominant formula every 4 h. Clinical examination is unremarkable.

Blood biochemistry is as follows:

Sodium	136 mmol/l
Potassium	4.1 mmol/l
Urea	1.4 mmol/l
Creatinine	42 µmol/l
Bicarbonate	22 mmol/l
Chloride	98 mmol/l

a What investigation would you perform?
b What would you advise her parents?

ANSWERS

a Salicylate poisoning. **1**
b Salicylate levels;
  Blood gases;
  Serum electrolytes.
c Treatment consists of bicarbonate replacement, rehydration and correction of electrolyte abnormalities.

Discussion

This child is hyperventilating and has a metabolic acidosis. In salicylate poisoning the only signs, particularly in infants, may be hyperventilation and dehydration. It is important to measure salicylate levels immediately and plot and repeat until the child is improving clinically. Electrolyte imbalance should be treated and potassium levels should be monitored carefully. A forced alkaline diuresis has little effect if there is satisfactory alkalinization and may aggravate pulmonary oedema. In severe cases haemodialysis may be required.

References

Forfar and Arneil's Textbook of Paediatrics 1782
Nelson's Textbook of Paediatrics 427, 2016–8

a Coeliac disease. **2**
b Jejunal biopsy.
c Malabsorption, poor dietary intake of iron.

Discussion

Coeliac disease is a gluten-induced enteropathy of uncertain aetiology. The prevalence is approximately 1 in 2000 in the UK, with a higher incidence in Ireland and a lower incidence outside Europe. Ten percent of patients have an affected first-degree relative and there is an association with HLA groups B8, DR3, DQw2, DR7 and DR2G.

Clinical features include buttock wasting, abdominal pain and distention, anorexia and vomiting. Stools are loose, pale, bulky and offensive. Iron deficiency anaemia is a frequent finding and folate levels may also be reduced.

Diagnosis is based on characteristic findings on jejunal biopsy — subtotal villus atrophy with crypt hypertrophy. There should be a marked clinical improvement on a gluten-free diet. The presence of antibodies to gliadin, reticulin and endomesium is of value for screening and for detecting relapse and non-compliance.

References

Forfar and Arneil's Textbook of Paediatrics 507–9
Nelson's Textbook of Paediatrics 1095–6

3

a Restrictive impairment.
b Pleural effusion secondary to pneumonia.
c Guillain–Barré;
  Duchenne muscular dystrophy;
  Kyphoscoliosis;
  Fibrosing alveolitis.

Discussion

FVC is the maximum volume of gas exhaled after a maximal inspiration. FEV1 is the maximum volume exhaled in the first second following maximum inspiration. The FEV1/FVC ratio represents the proportion of the vital capacity that can be exhaled in the first second. In this case both the FVC and FEV1 are significantly reduced thus indicating that there are functionally small lungs. Due to the symmetrical reduction in both parameters the FEV1/FVC ratio remains unaltered. Examples of restrictive lung parenchymal disease include conditions where the interstitium is filled with fluid (oedema or infection), alveolar collapse or destruction. Neuromuscular disease, congenital malformations or abdominal distension can all cause restriction of chest wall movement with a similar effect on FEV1/FVC.

Pleural effusion complicating pneumonia is more common with staphylococcal infections. As this boy had not improved clinically after 2 days of treatment with intravenous penicillin, anti-staphylococcal agents should be added and drainage considered. If drainage is difficult intrapleural streptokinase may have a role to help dissolve the fibrin clots.

References
Forfar and Arneil's Textbook of Paediatrics 573, 642, 1384
Nelson's Textbook of Paediatrics 1170–5, 1184–5

4

a Wilson's disease.
b Kayer–Fleischer rings.
c Serum copper and caeruloplasmin levels may be reduced;
Urinary copper levels will be elevated;
Penicillamine load;
Liver biopsy.

Discussion

ANSWERS

Wilson's disease is an autosomal recessive disease which is characterized by defective biliary copper excretion. Copper accumulates in various tissues including liver, brain, eyes and kidneys. Clinical features include hepatosplenomegaly, jaundice, cirrhosis, portal hypertension, gall-stones, renal tubular acidosis and Kayer–Fleischer rings. In adolescence it commonly presents with intellectual deterioration and progressive extrapyramidal signs. Almost always an element of Fanconi's syndrome is present — hence the glycosuria. Diagnosis may be difficult as 24% have normal caeruloplasmin levels. Other diagnostic tests include a penicillamine load which causes an increase in urinary copper. A liver biopsy in the early stages shows glycogen nuclei and Mallory bodies, but in the later stages it is indistinguishable from other causes of macronodular cirrhosis. The aim of treatment is to lower tissue copper levels. Those with a milder form of the disease may respond to a low copper diet (high levels of copper are found in shellfish, liver, broccoli, nuts and chocolate), and treatment with penicillamine, a copper chelating agent. Those with advanced disease at the time of diagnosis may require a liver transplant. Liver transplantation, if successful, reverses the biochemical abnormalities.

References
Forfar and Arneil's Textbook of Paediatrics 554–5, 1213–4, 1754
Nelson's Textbook of Paediatrics 1139–40

5
    a Age 6–7 years.
    b Minor dysmorphic signs.
    c This boy is unlikely to have a specific medical diagnosis but fragile X should be excluded.

Discussion
From the Griffiths Mental Development Scales in year 8, one would expect a boy to accurately draw a diamond, be able to count backwards from 20, know 'heavy' and 'light', know 6–7 coins, and say three digits backwards.

The incidence of fragile X is approximately 1 per 1000 males. Developmental ability varies but most have moderate to severe developmental delay. Other features include large head and forehead, long ears, prominent chin and macro-orchidism after puberty.

References
Forfar and Arneil's Textbook of Paediatrics 69–70
Nelson's Textbook of Paediatrics 318–9
Griffiths Mental Development Scales (R. Griffiths), Test Agency Ltd, High Wycombe, UK

6
    a Duchenne muscular dystrophy.

ANSWERS

b Gower's sign;
   Calf hypertrophy.
c Muscle biopsy;
   DNA analysis.

Discussion

Duchenne muscular dystrophy is inherited as a sex-linked recessive condition, with the abnormality in the region of Xp21. Presentation of the disease is usually between the ages of 1 and 4 years with a history of delayed walking, frequent falls, difficulty climbing stairs or getting up from the floor. After falling, 'climbing up the legs' is character-istic—this is known as Gower's sign. Other features in-clude calf hypertrophy, waddling gait, toe walking and tightening of the tendo Achilles. The creatine phosphokinase (CPK) levels are very high initially but as muscle fibres are replaced by fat and fibrous tissue, the CPK levels fall.

A muscle biopsy is required to confirm the diagnosis. Referral to a geneticist for DNA analysis is recommended and antenatal diagnosis offered in future pregnancies.

References

Forfar and Arneil's Textbook of Paediatrics 794–7
Nelson's Textbook of Paediatrics 1671–2, 1746–8

a Urine—orotic acid;   **7**
   Blood—amino acids.
b Ornithine transcarbamylase deficiency (OTC).
c Low protein diet;
   Sodium benzoate.

Discussion

The important points of note here are that there is hyperammonaemia; that the male baby had a male sibling who died in the first week; that there is no acidosis and that the baby suddenly collapsed in the absence of sepsis or liver abnormalities (e.g. Reye's syndrome). This baby shows symptoms of hyperammonaemia, i.e. vomiting, agitation, seizures and episodes of decreased consciousness. Hyperammonaemia with acidosis occurs in organic acidaemias, hyperammonaemia with no acidosis occurs in urea cycle disorders. OTC deficiency is probably the most common urea cycle disorder; it is an X-linked dominant disorder where the male offspring are severely affected. Blood ammonia is grossly elevated as are glutamine and alanine. The 'gold standard' test is measurement of orotic acid in the urine — this is markedly elevated.

Once the baby is stabilized initially, the hyperammonia can be treated with sodium benzoate as an infusion. Occasionally babies need peritoneal dialysis. It is important that the future diet is very low in protein. Citrulline and phenylbutyrate have also been given in the long term to control the blood ammonia.

References
Forfar and Arneil's Textbook of Paediatrics 1183
Nelson's Textbook of Paediatrics 351–3

8

a Wiskott–Aldrich syndrome.
b Inheritance is X-linked recessive.
c Coombs-positive haemolytic anaemia.

Discussion
Wiskott–Aldrich syndrome is characterized by the triad of thrombocytopenia, eczema and immunodeficiency. The condition often presents in the first 3 months of life with bruising and bleeding. An eczematous rash develops and the child may suffer from recurrent infections with opportunistic pathogens and herpes infections.

Treatment is supportive. Platelet transfusions may be required for bleeding episodes and topical steroids for the eczema. Intravenous immunoglobins may be given but despite these supportive treatments, the prognosis is poor. Bone marrow transplantation may be considered the ideal option.

References
Forfar and Arneil's Textbook of Paediatrics 1315–6
Nelson's Textbook of Paediatrics 576

a Shortened PR interval — approximately 0.08 s.   **9**
b Wolff–Parkinson–White syndrome.
c An echocardiogram.

Discussion

Wolff–Parkinson–White syndrome is usually associated with normal cardiac structure but may also be associated with Ebstein anomaly, cardiomyopathy and corrected transposition. There is a shortened PR interval (normally 0.12–0.2 seconds or 3–5 small squares). There is a marginally increased QRS complex and the slow upstroke of the QRS is the delta wave.

References
Forfar and Arneil's Textbook of Paediatrics 697
Nelson's Textbook of Paediatrics 1340

a Angelman's syndrome.   **10**
b Prader–Willi.

Discussion

The term 'imprinting' describes the phenomenon whereby certain genes function differently, depending on whether they are paternally or maternally inherited. This is illustrated by deletions in the q11–13 region of chromosome 15, which results in either Prader–Willi if paternally derived, or Angelman's syndrome if the deletion is on the maternally derived chromosome. In patients with Prader–Willi syndrome with no chromosomal deletion, both chromosome 15's are maternally inherited. This phenomenon is called uniparental disomy.

ANSWERS

Features of Prader–Willi syndrome include a history of poor fetal movements *in utero*, feeding difficulties and hypotonia in the newborn period. Characteristic facial features include a carp-like mouth, a narrow forehead and an anti-mongolian slant to the eyes. There is hypogonadism and despite the early poor feeding an insatiable appetite develops later and this combined with very low energy requirements and inactivity leads to gross obesity. Scoliosis may develop and this combined with obesity may lead to respiratory failure and premature death.

Features of Angelman's syndrome include microcephaly, developmental delay, ataxia, absent speech and epilepsy.

References

ABC of Clinical Genetics (ed. H. Kingston), 2nd edn, 1997. BMA, London, 8–9

Forfar and Arneil's Textbook of Paediatrics 67, 1158, 1289

Nelson's Textbook of Paediatrics 311, 320

---

11 a Reassurance that this is normal premenstrual discharge.
b No further investigations are needed.

Discussion

That this is normal premenstrual discharge is supported by the fact that there is no sign of inflammation and there are no white cells. When a girl enters puberty, the vaginal pH falls due to increased production of acetic and lactic acids, with increased superficial cell proliferation and enhancement of normal vaginal flora. Antibiotics are not indicated and may lead to thrush. Oestrogen creams which are sometimes helpful in the prepubertal child are not helpful—this girl is producing her own oestrogens. Other vaginal creams and tampons should be discouraged.

Reference

Nelson's Textbook of Paediatrics 1555

ANSWERS

a Atrial septal defect.

12

b Surgical correction in childhood.

Discussion

Children with atrial septal defects are usually asymptomatic, unless the defect is large. On auscultation there is wide splitting of the second sound, with no variation with respiration. Murmurs are due to high flow across the tricuspid and pulmonary valves and not through the septal defect itself.

The chest X-ray shows cardiomegaly with an enlarged right atrium and pulmonary plethora. The ECG shows sinus rhythm, with normal axis in ostium secundum defects or sinus venous defects and left axis deviation in ostium primum defects. An RSR' pattern is seen in the right chest leads. This is not incomplete bundle branch block, there is no delay in conduction in the right bundle branch and the RSR' pattern probably represents prolonged depolarization of a hypertrophied right ventricle. This pattern is seen in others with a hypertrophied right ventricle of varying aetiology and in 5–10% of normal children and is therefore not pathognomonic for atrial septal defects.

It is unusual for secundum defects to close spontaneously. Long-term results following surgery are excellent but persistent right ventricular enlargement, arrhythmias and conduction defects occur.

References

Forfar and Arneil's Textbook of Paediatrics 674–5
Nelson's Textbook of Paediatrics 1288–92

a Serum IgE antibodies;

13

  Chest X-ray;
  Blood and sputum culture.
b Allergic aspergillosis.

Discussion

This boy was obviously well controlled with regards to the recurrent *Pseudomonas aeruginosa* infection. These acute symptoms indicate a new infection and fit with aspergillosis. This complication presents usually with wheezing, increased cough, fever and profound breathlessness. There may also be rust-coloured sputum. Chest X-ray may reveal interstitial infiltrates. The diagnosis is substantiated by finding *Aspergillus* in fresh sputum or an elevated IgE level. The prognosis is generally very good, with corticosteroids being used to reduce inflammation.

References
Forfar and Arneil's Textbook of Paediatrics 630, 1376
Nelson's Textbook of Paediatrics 1248

---

14 a Langerhans cell histiocytosis, stage 3.
   b Skin biopsy;
      Skeletal survey;
      Urea and electrolytes, liver function tests;
      Bone marrow biopsy.
   c Steroids and chemotherapy.

Discussion

Langerhans cell histiocytosis (class 1 histiocytosis) results from a proliferation of Langerhans cells, probably secondary to a defect in immunoregulation. The most useful marker to distinguish Langerhans cells is the presence of Birkbeck granules. Classification is according to stage of bone and organ involvement. In stage 1 there is a single lytic lesion, stage 2 multiple lytic lesions, stage 3A bone plus soft tissue lesions often with diabetes insipidus and stage 3B disseminated soft tissue lesions.

Treatment for stages 1 and 2 involves excision of the boney lesion and irradiation for lesions which cannot be reached. For stage 3 the treatment depends on the degree of organ involvement, but initial treatment is with steroids, moving on to chemotherapy (single therapy and then combination therapy) if control is not achieved.

This baby had bone and soft tissue involvement, therefore stage 3 disease.

References

Forfar and Arneil's Textbook of Paediatrics 1002, 1726
Nelson's Textbook of Paediatrics 1997–9

---

a No—this is a grade 3 reaction and suggests the possibility of active tuberculosis. He should have further investigations including a chest X-ray. **15**
b Meningococcal vaccine;
  Typhoid vaccine;
  Yellow fever vaccination certificate is required from travellers coming from infected areas.

Discussion

Individuals over 3 months of age should have a tuberculin test prior to BCG immunization. The greater the strength of reaction to the test the greater the chance that the individual has active tuberculosis. The Heaf reaction is graded 0–4, grade 0 is where there is no induration at the puncture site and grade 4 is where there is solid induration over 10 mm wide.

The meningococcal vaccine is effective against *Neisseria meningitidis* serotype A and C organisms. Routine immunization is not recommended in the UK as the risk of meningococcal disease is very low, and those cases which do occur are usually due to Group B organisms, for which there is as yet no available vaccine. The vaccine is specifically recommended for close contacts of cases of Group A or C meningitis, for use to control local outbreaks and for travel to high-risk areas. Immunization is recommended for travel to Bhutan, Sub-Saharan Africa, Delhi and Pakistan.

ANSWERS

References

Immunisation Against Infectious Disease (eds D.M. Salisbury & N.T. Begg), 1996. HMSO, London, 150–2, 225, 231–2

Forfar and Arneil's Textbook of Paediatrics 1348, 1394–5

Nelson's Textbook of Paediatrics 770–1, 845–6

---

16   a Complement levels;
ASO titre;
Renal biopsy;
Immune complex measurements;
IgA levels.

b IgA nephritis (Berger's nephropathy).

Discussion

The renal function is normal despite the haematuria. It is very tempting to immediately think of post-streptococcal glomerulonephritis with the sore throats but this is associated with renal insufficiency as well as oedema and hypertension.

IgA nephritis is one of the most common causes of gross haematuria. IgA is deposited in the mesangium, the biopsies show focal and segmental proliferation. The renal function normally remains relatively normal and protein excretion below 1 g/24 h. A small number progress to end-stage renal failure.

References

Forfar and Arneil's Textbook of Paediatrics 1049–51

Nelson's Textbook of Paediatrics 1485

---

17   a Congenital myotonic dystrophy.

b EMG;
Muscle biopsy;
DNA analysis;
Shake mothers hand.

Discussion

Dystrophia myotonica is inherited in an autosomal dominant fashion with variable penetrance. Many mothers with the condition do not actually realize that they have it until their child is diagnosed. Polyhydramnios may result secondary to swallowing problems in the fetus and tube feeding is often required in the first weeks of life. Resuscitation may be required at birth and ventilation may be necessary due to diaphragmatic abnormalities. Children have hypotonia with characteristic myopathic facies. Moderate learning difficulties are common but intelligence may be normal. Muscle biopsy shows small type 1 muscle fibres with elevated acid phosphatase levels. DNA analysis should be offered—the gene locus is on the long arm of chromosome 19. The mother may have difficulties trying to relax her grip after shaking hands, with rapid flexion and extension of the fingers. An EMG of the small muscles of the hand will reveal 'dive bomber' myotonic discharges.

References

Forfar and Arneil's Textbook of Paediatrics 798–9
Nelson's Textbook of Paediatrics 1750

a A banded karyotype illustrating a female trisomy 18.
b Prominent occiput, low set ears, clinodactyly, rocker-bottom feet, hypoplastic nails, micrognathia and low birth weight.
c An echocardiogram and renal ultrasound to help determine prognosis as cardiac and renal abnormalities are common.

Discussion

Trisomy 18 (Edward's syndrome) has an incidence of approximately 0.12 per 1000 live births. Most cases are due to maternal non-disjunction and there is an increasing incidence with maternal age. The risk of recurrence is low unless there is a parental balanced translocation. Usually affected infants only survive for a few weeks or months but there have been a few reported cases where there has been survival into the teenage years.

References
Forfar and Arneil's Textbook of Paediatrics 63–4
Nelson's Textbook of Paediatrics 315–6, 1682

---

19 a Inconclusive as not enough sweat obtained.
b Repeat the sweat test.

Discussion
Children with cystic fibrosis have elevated sweat sodium and chloride levels but for valid interpretation of sweat test results, at least 100 mg of sweat needs to be collected, otherwise results are meaningless. If a repeat sweat test is normal, further investigations should be considered, e.g. measurement of immunoglobulin levels, electron microscopy of nasal cilia. If the sweat test results are characteristic of cystic fibrosis, genetic testing may then be performed.

References
Forfar and Arneil's Textbook of Paediatrics 626–7
Nelson's Textbook of Paediatrics 1243

---

20 a Aortic stenosis.
b He should avoid competitive sport;
Antibiotic prophylaxis should be given for dental treatment.

Discussion
Echocardiography is used to look at the site of stenosis and Doppler studies or cardiac catheterization may be used to assess the severity. Most children with aortic stenosis are asymptomatic although those with severe obstruction may have syncope, shortness of breath or angina on exertion. Sudden death, although rare, may

occur during stressful exercise and therefore competitive sport should be avoided. On clinical examination the presence of an ejection systolic click loudest over the apex or left sternal border is characteristic of valvular stenosis with a pliable valve. As the severity of obstruction increases the sound of the aortic valve closing becomes softer and delayed and the second heart sound becomes single or shows paradoxical splitting.

In subvalvular or supravalvular stenosis, there is no click and a soft diastolic murmur is suggestive of aortic regurgitation.

References
Forfar and Arneil's Textbook of Paediatrics 679
Nelson's Textbook of Paediatrics 1300–1

---

a Gilbert's syndrome. **21**
b No treatment is necessary.

Discussion
Gilbert's syndrome refers to a mild unconjugated hyper-bilirubinaemia in the absence of overt haemolysis or liver disease. In most cases there is diminished activity of specific hepatic enzymes which suggests a defect in glucuronidation. An autosomal dominant mode of inheritance has been suggested. The prognosis is excellent, with no evidence that it is associated with more serious conditions. In this case the family needs reassurance and the headaches need to be investigated further if they persist.

References
Forfar and Arneil's Textbook of Paediatrics 1212
Nelson's Textbook of Paediatrics 1036

---

a This shows a chaotic pattern of high voltage, slow wave **22** activity. It is referred to as hypsarrhythmia.
b Infantile spasms.

Discussion

Hypsarrhythmia typically illustrates the clinical condition of infantile spasms. These usually begin between the ages of 4 and 8 months and are characterized by brief symmetric contractions of the limbs, trunk and head. The sudden 'fling' forward is often referred to as a 'Salaam attack'. The spasms occur in 'volleys' with only seconds in between each one. They often occur when the child is drowsy.

Approximately 80% of infantile spasms are related to prenatal, perinatal or postnatal events, e.g. hypoxic ischaemic encephalopathy, congenital or postnatal infections, metabolic disorders and head injury. There is a high risk of developmental delay in this group (approximately 80–90%). There are a minority who have 'cryptogenic' infantile spasms where there is no underlying cause—the outlook for this group is very good.

References

Forfar and Arneil's Textbook of Paediatrics 755–8
Nelson's Textbook of Paediatrics 1690

---

23 a Infectious mononucleosis.
   b Monospot test/Paul Bunnell test.

Discussion

Infectious mononucleosis results from infection with the Epstein–Barr virus. Moderate lymphocytosis and atypical mononuclear cells are found. Autoimmune haemolytic anaemia, Reye's syndrome, splenic rupture and CNS involvement may all occur. A macular rash occurs in > 90% of individuals if ampicillin is given.

References

Forfar and Arneil's Textbook of Paediatrics 939
Nelson's Textbook of Paediatrics 897–901

ANSWERS

a Syndrome of inappropriate secretion of anti-diuretic **24**
  hormone (SIADH).
b Perinatal hypoxia/ischaemia.
c Fluid restriction to 50–75% of normal requirements.

Discussion

SIADH in the newborn period is associated with birth asphyxia, respiratory distress syndrome or intraventricular haemorrhage. In older children it occurs in association with meningitis, encephalitis or central nervous system tumours. It may also complicate pneumonia, burns, trauma or chemotherapy. Biochemical findings include dilutional hyponatraemia and hypo-osmolality. At first signs and symptoms are due to the underlying problem and then vomiting, convulsions and coma occur.

References

Forfar and Arneil's Textbook of Paediatrics 286, 480, 1111–12
Nelson's Textbook of Paediatrics 215, 1576–7

a X-linked dominant. **25**
b Vitamin D-resistant rickets.

Discussion

An X-linked dominant gene will give rise to the disorder in both hemizygous males and heterozygous females. An affected male transmits the disease to all of his daughters and none of his sons. Fifty per cent of both daughters and sons of affected females will be affected. In some disorders the condition is lethal in the hemizygous male (e.g. incontinentia pigmenti).

References

Forfar and Arneil's Textbook of Paediatrics 74
Nelson's Textbook of Paediatrics 310

ANSWERS

26   a Congenital hypothyroidism.

       b Treatment is with L-thyroxine 10 μmol/kg/day.

Discussion

Infants are usually asymptomatic at birth, but develop symptoms including prolonged jaundice, umbilical hernias, constipation, hypothermia, oedema, feeding difficulties and lethargy if left untreated. Treatment is with thyroxine and the dose should be adjusted to maintain a 'near normal' TSH level. Treatment is for life.

References

Forfar and Arneil's Textbook of Paediatrics 1118–9
Nelson's Textbook of Paediatrics 1589–94

---

27   a Neuroblastoma.

       b VMA levels;

         Localization of tumour by non-invasive techniques, e.g. abdominal ultrasound, MIBG scan (^{123}I-metaiodobenzyl guanidine).

Discussion

Neuroblastomas arise from neural crest cells. The most common primary site is the adrenal gland, other sites being within the abdomen, the chest, pelvis and neck. Presentation is often with an abdominal mass, accompanied by features of marrow infiltration, e.g. bruising, anaemia, irritability and fever. Seventy per cent of children have metastases at the time of diagnosis, and periorbital bruising is suggestive of disease within the orbit or sphenoidal bone. Eighty-five to 90% of tumours have elevated levels of catecholamine in the serum and urine and measurement of vanillyl mandelic acid (VMA) levels and homovanillic acid (HVA) levels can be used to monitor treatment. The MIBG scan is used to identify tumour deposits and is more useful than bone scanning. There is a

ANSWERS

neuroblastoma staging system — stages 1, 2A, 2B, 3, 4 and 4S. Good prognostic features include age <1 year, stages 1, 2 and 4S, primary tumour in the neck and thorax and a low serum ferritin level. Chemotherapy is the main form of treatment but complete resection should be attempted for stages 1 and 2.

References
Forfar and Arneil's Textbook of Paediatrics 984–7
Nelson's Textbook of Paediatrics 1460–3

---

a Non-ketotic hyperglycinaemia.   **28**
b The condition is usually fatal in those with a neonatal presentation.

Discussion
In this condition there is a defect in glycine cleavage. Apnoeas, seizures and coma are common and result in death in the neonatal period. Infants who survive have myoclonus, failure to thrive, microcephaly and severe learning difficulties.

Investigations reveal an elevated urine and CSF glycine level and plasma glycine is usually but not invariably elevated. Neutropenia and hyperammonia may occur and the EEG may show hypsarrhythmia.

References
Forfar and Arneil's Textbook of Paediatrics 1185
Nelson's Textbook of Paediatrics 345–7
Roberton's Textbook of Neonatology 831

---

a Hereditary spherocytosis.   **29**
b Autosomal dominant with variable expression.
c Treatment involves splenectomy (in severe cases), prophylactic penicillin, folic acid and polyvalent pneumococcal vaccine (given prior to splenectomy).

Discussion

In hereditary spherocytosis, red blood cells become convex instead of the normal biconcave configuration. The diagnosis is made from the increased osmotic fragility of red cells or from a positive family history. Clinical features include anaemia and jaundice of fluctuating severity. Haemolysis may be exacerbated with intercurrent infections. Pigment gall-stones are common and parvovirus infection or folate deficiency may precipitate an aplastic crisis.

References

Forfar and Arneil's Textbook of Paediatrics 250, 928–9
Nelson's Textbook of Paediatrics 1392–4

---

30 a Renal tubular acidosis—distal type.
  b Urinary pH;
     Urinary excretion of glucose, phosphate and amino acids.

Discussion

The results show hypokalaemia and hyperchloraemia with nephrocalcinosis. A urinary pH of <6 in the presence of systemic acidosis will confirm the diagnosis. Looking at urinary excretion will help distinguish proximal from distal renal tubular acidosis. Proximal renal tubular acidosis is associated with glycosuria, phosphaturia and aminoaciduria.

References

Forfar and Arneil's Textbook of Paediatrics 289–90, 1030
Nelson's Textbook of Paediatrics 1504–6

---

31 a Glycogen storage disease (Von Gierke disease—type 1).
  b Liver biopsy and glucose-6-phosphatase assay.
  c Normal cerebral development should occur providing prolonged periods of hypoglycaemia are avoided.

ANSWERS

Discussion

This baby exhibits a metabolic acidosis, hyperlipidaemia, hypoglycaemia and hepatomegaly. These findings fit with a glycogen storage disease. Type 1a describes an abnormality of the enzyme glucose 6-phosphatase and primarily affects the liver, kidney and intestines.

References

Forfar and Arneil's Textbook of Paediatrics 1216–7
Nelson's Textbook of Paediatrics 391, 393

---

a Renal failure secondary to vitamin supplementation **32** (vitamin D).

b Plain X-ray—nephrolithiasis.

Discussion

Vitamin D toxicity is associated with loss of appetite, nausea, vomiting and constipation and hypercalcaemia, which may be associated with thirst and polyuria. Nephrocalcinosis and renal failure may also occur. Treatment of toxicity includes glucocorticoid administration which gradually reduces intestinal calcium absorption, a low calcium diet and stopping vitamin D supplementation.

References

Forfar and Arneil's Textbook of Paediatrics 1268
Nelson's Textbook of Paediatrics 183–4

---

a Mitral stenosis. **33**

b Lying in the left lateral position listening with the bell of the stethoscope;
The murmur may be accentuated by exercise.

Discussion

The normal pressure in the right atrium is approximately

ANSWERS

3 mmHg, in the right ventricle approximately 25/3, and in the pulmonary artery approximately 25/10. The oxygen saturation throughout the right side should be around 75% and the saturation throughout the left side should not fall below 95%. The pressure in the left atrium should be around 8 mmHg, in the left ventricle 100/8 mmHg and in the aorta approximately 100/60 mmHg.

In this case the saturation throughout the right side is low while the pressures are high. The left atrial pressure is also high, whilst the left ventricular pressure is normal. Tying this together with a history of fatigue and a murmur on auscultation, the data are consistent with a diagnosis of mitral stenosis. In mitral stenosis there is a loud first sound, an opening snap and a low-pitched rumbling diastolic murmur. Congenital mitral stenosis is relatively rare with congestive cardiac failure and cyanosis generally occurring within the first 2 years. Mitral stenosis may be secondary to rheumatic fever, the mitral valve being the valve most commonly affected in this condition.

References
Forfar and Arneil's Textbook of Paediatrics 701
Nelson's Textbook of Paediatrics 1304

---

34   a No treatment is needed.
   b Breast milk jaundice.

Discussion
Breast feeding has many advantages for the baby and should be promoted. Advantages include optimal nutrient content, and reduced risk of allergies and infection. Although breast feeding may result in a prolonged unconjugated hyperbilirubinaemia, this usually disappears by the age of 6 weeks. Stopping breast feeding may cause a reduction in bilirubin, but continued breast feeding should be encouraged. Other causes of persistent unconjugated

hyperbilirubinaemia include hypothyroidism, intestinal stasis and haemolytic anaemias.

References
Forfar and Arneil's Textbook of Paediatrics 244, 364
Nelson's Textbook of Paediatrics 493–6

---

a Hyperinflation;   **35**
Obstructive airways disease;
Partial reversibility.
b Plethysmography;
Helium dilution.

Discussion
Looking at these results the main disparities are that the residual volume (that is the volume of gas in the lungs after maximum expiration) is much greater than predicted suggesting hyperinflation. The FEV1 value increases following salbutamol indicating a degree of reversibility. The FEV1/FVC ratio is 0.6 (60%) which indicates moderate to severe obstructive disease.

Plethysmography and helium dilution are techniques used to measure total lung volume. Plethysmography uses the principles of Boyle's law to measure the total volume of gas in the thoracic cage. The helium dilution technique depends on the equilibration between gas in the lungs and a helium/air mixture, but gives less accurate results than the former technique.

References
Forfar and Arneil's Textbook of Paediatrics 575–7
Nelson's Textbook of Paediatrics 1172

---

a This suggests a diagnosis of mosaic Turner's   **36**
syndrome.
b Low hairline, short webbed neck, shield-shaped chest,

ANSWERS

widely spaced nipples and increased carrying angle at the elbows.

c Cardiac screening—coarctation of the aorta occurs in Turner's syndrome;
Renal ultrasound—renal abnormalities associated with Turner's syndrome include horseshoe kidneys and duplex ureters.

Discussion

Mosaicism refers to the presence of two or more cell lines, differing in chromosomal constitution, but which derive from a single zygote. Chromosomal mosaicism arises by postzygotic errors in mitosis. In this case, one cell line is 45X suggesting Turner's syndrome and the other cell line has a normal female karyotype 46XX. The diagnosis is therefore mosaic Turner's syndrome. Sixty percent of Turner's syndrome cases have a 45XO karyotype, 15% have the mosaic form XX/XO, 10% have an isochromosome Xp or Xq and the remaining 15% have other chromosomal abnormalities, e.g. 46Xdel(X).

References

Forfar and Arneil's Textbook of Paediatrics 67–8
Nelson's Textbook of Paediatrics 317–8, 1635–6

37

a Type 2 gynaecomastia.

b Drugs—marijuana, anabolic steroids, opiates, amphetamines;
Medications—digoxin, spironolactone, antihypertensives, oestrogens;
Medical conditions—testicular failure, thyroid disease, gonadal tumours, androgen insensitivity syndrome, Klinefelter's syndrome, hyperprolactinaemia.

c Counselling;
Surgery (subareolar mastectomy) may be considered if there are major psychological problems and the condition persists.

ANSWERS

Discussion

Type 1 gynaecomastia occurs in 60% of boys mid-puberty (puberty rating 2–4); it is usually less than 3 cm in diameter and resolves in under 2 years.

Type 2 gynaecomastia occurs in later puberty and is greater than 3 cm in diameter; it too may spontaneously resolve but if it has persisted for more than 3 years it is unlikely to, and therefore surgical resection may be offered if the psychological effects are interfering with quality of life.

Enquiry into illicit drug use is important—this young man had started using anabolic steroids at the local gym, hence the small testicular volume.

References

Forfar and Arneil's Textbook of Paediatrics 440
Nelson's Textbook of Paediatrics 60, 556

38

a 90.
b 769.
c 84%.

Discussion

This question requires some knowledge of the properties of a normal distribution and the proportions under the curve (Fig. 16). As almost all human measurements follow a normal distribution, this is not an unreasonable question!

a 24.8 is two standard deviations above the mean and therefore 2% fall above this—2% of 500 is 10; 12.2 is one standard deviation below the mean and 16% of the population will be below this—16% of 500 is 80. Adding these figures together (10 + 80) gives an answer of 90.

b 29.0 g/dl is three standard deviations from the mean and only 0.13% will exceed this value. A population of 769 (100/0.13) is required before it would be expected

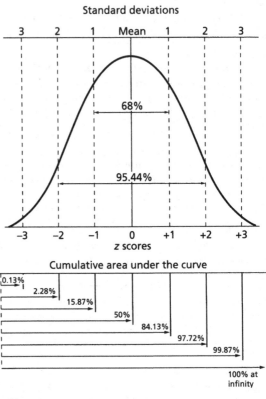

Standard deviations

Cumulative area under the curve

Fig. 16

to include an individual with a value three standard deviations above the mean.

c A value of 20.6 g/dl is one standard deviation from the mean and in a normal distribution 68% lie between −1.0 standard deviations and +1.0 standard deviations from the mean. Sixteen percent will have values < −1.0 standard deviations from the mean. The answer is therefore 16% + 68% = 84%.

References
Nelson's Textbook of Paediatrics 8, 72
Basic Epidemiology (eds R. Beaglehole, R. Bonita & T. Kjellström), 1993. WHO Publications, 59–62

a The anaesthetic drugs have caused peripheral vasodilation resulting in a cyanotic spell. This has been exacerbated by hypovolaemia due to preoperative fasting.

b Oxygen;
Intravenous morphine;
Volume replacement;
Propranolol;
Other vasoconstrictors (e.g. methoxamine).

Discussion

Tetralogy of Fallot classically consists of the combination of right ventricular outflow obstruction (pulmonary stenosis), ventricular septal defect, 'overlying aorta' and subsequent right ventricular hypertrophy. Cyanosis is most obvious as the outflow obstruction becomes more marked. Hypercyanotic attacks occur when there is either increased resistance in the right ventricular outflow or a transient decrease in the systemic resistance (as in this case). In this severe case, morphine should be given immediately (if the child was not ventilated then O_2 should also be given). β-adrenergic blockade has been successfully given particularly where there is tachycardia, and drugs that increase systemic resistance, such as methoxamine, will also decrease the right to left shunt.

References

Forfar and Arneil's Textbook of Paediatrics 688–90
Nelson's Textbook of Paediatrics 1311–5

a Kawasaki disease.
b Aneurysms — especially of the coronary arteries.
c Gammaglobulin, aspirin.

Discussion

Kawasaki disease presents as an acute febrile illness, predominantly in children under 5 years of age. The condition is characterized by fever, conjunctivitis, mucous membrane changes, erythema, oedema and desquamation of the palms and soles, polymorphous rash and cervical lymphadenopathy. Associated features include arthritis, irritability, diarrhoea and abdominal pain, pericarditis and myocarditis. Aneurysms, including coronary artery aneurysms, may occur and must be considered.

The platelet count is usually normal in the first week, rising in the second and third weeks. The white blood count is usually elevated in the first week with a neutrophilia and later a lymphocytosis occurs. The ESR and C reactive protein are usually elevated. Gammaglobulin, if given during the initial illness, reduces the risk of coronary artery aneurysms. Low dose aspirin may be given for its anti-inflammatory action and activity against platelet aggregation, for a 6–8 week period.

References

Forfar and Arneil's Textbook of Paediatrics 1536–8
Nelson's Textbook of Paediatrics 678–80

41
a A liver biopsy would confirm the diagnosis but clotting derangements must be corrected first.
b Reye's syndrome.

Discussion

Reye's syndrome is a rare, acute encephalopathy. It usually occurs during a viral illness or exanthema (10% of cases are secondary to chickenpox) and there is an association with aspirin. It is characterized by an abnormality of mitochondrial structure and function, particularly in the liver. The diagnosis should be suspected where there is encephalopathy with evidence of liver involvement such as hypoglycaemia, elevated liver enzymes or ammonia levels or prolonged PTT. A liver biopsy reveals swollen mitochondria with reduced mitochondrial enzyme levels and normal cytoplasmic enzyme activity. Management involves the control of raised intracranial pressure, correction of hypovolaemia and maintenance of blood sugar. An 'acute liver failure' regime may be required with the use of lactulose, cimetidine and vitamin K.

References

Forfar and Arneil's Textbook of Paediatrics 553, 1182, 1416
Nelson's Textbook of Paediatrics 1144–5

---

a Visual acuity/visual fields/ophthalmoscopy.   **42**
b Drug ingestion.
c Benign intracranial hypertension (pseudotumour cerebri).
d No treatment if mild, steroids if reduced visual acuity. Lumbar punctures may be performed to reduce CSF pressure.

Discussion

Benign intracranial hypertension is a rare cause of headaches and generally warrants thorough neuroradiological investigation to exclude small central tumours, e.g. craniopharyngiomas. Benign intracranial hypertension may occur secondary to hypoparathyroidism, galactosaemia, steroid therapy withdrawal, tetracycline and high dose vitamin A. This boy was on tetracycline for his acne. Damage to the optic nerve is of immediate concern — hence the importance of visual acuity assessment. Benign intracranial hypertension usually subsides but relief of intracranial pressure by repeated lumbar punctures or steroids is sometimes indicated. Acetazolamide (sometimes given with a loop diuretic) may be required if there is an inadequate response to steroid therapy. If medical treatment fails surgical intervention may be required.

References

Forfar and Arneil's Textbook of Paediatrics 738–9
Nelson's Textbook of Paediatrics 174, 1735

ANSWERS

43   a Beta thalassaemia major.
    b Repeated transfusions to avoid the bone problems associated with compensatory marrow hyperplasia;
       Daily subcutaneous desferal;
       Oral vitamin C.
    c Hypersplenism;
       Growth impairment;
       Delayed puberty;
       Diabetes mellitus;
       Cardiac arrhythmias and heart failure.

Discussion

Children with thalassaemia major usually present in the first year of life. In beta thalassaemia major, no beta chains are produced and haemoglobin is predominantly in the form of Hb F. In the milder heterozygous beta thalassaemia, some Hb A is produced. The blood film shows many normoblasts but the reticulocyte count is only moderately raised due to dyserythropoiesis. Regular transfusion inevitably leads to iron in most of the body tissues resulting in secondary failure if desferroxime is not given with transfusions.

References

Forfar and Arneil's Textbook of Paediatrics 931–4
Nelson's Textbook of Paediatrics 1402–3

---

44   a *Chlamydia trachomatis, Ureaplasma urealyticum, Trichomonas vaginalis.*
    b History of sexual intercourse, including number of sexual partners.
    c Contact tracing.
    d Doxycycline.

Discussion

If his dysuria was secondary to a urinary tract infection, it is more likely that his urine sample would have tested positive for nitrites and blood (80% of urinary tract infections are caused by *E. coli*).

Contact tracing can be difficult as the incubation period can be up to 3 weeks and infections may be asymptomatic. Concurrent infections with other organisms need to be considered and single dose therapy given if compliance is thought to be a problem.

References

Forfar and Arneil's Textbook of Paediatrics 1073, 1451, 1459
Nelson's Textbook of Paediatrics 552–3

---

a Organic acidaemia.   **45**
b Intravenous fluids, antibiotics.
c Urine organic acids, toxicology screen, septic screen.

Discussion

The presentation of an underweight infant with a marked metabolic acidosis suggests an organic acidaemia but possible overwhelming infection needs to be treated. Diabetic ketoacidosis may present in this way but is rare in this age group compared with older children. Aminoacidopathies rarely present with marked acidosis. Poisoning needs to be considered and often a toxic screen is forgotten in the height of resuscitation.

References

Forfar and Arneil's Textbook of Paediatrics 1188–9
Nelson's Textbook of Paediatrics 340–5

---

a Patent ductus arteriosus.   **46**
b Attention to fluid balance to prevent fluid retention;
   Haemoglobin measurement and correction of anaemia
   if applicable;
   Course of indomethacin.

c Indomethacin may cause clotting abnormalities and subsequent bleeding. It may also cause oliguria, renal failure, gut/cerebral ischaemia.

Discussion
Other features of patent ductus arteriosus in the preterm infant include apnoea, hypertension, heart failure, metabolic acidosis and cardiomegaly. If there is a contraindication to indomethacin or its treatment proves unsuccessful, surgical ligation may be required. Complications of PDA include endarteritis, congestive cardiac failure and the development of pulmonary vascular disease.

References
Forfar and Arneil's Textbook of Paediatrics 227–8
Nelson's Textbook of Paediatrics 483–4, 1295–6

---

47 a 333.3 per 1000 (33%).
b 166.7 per 1000 (16.7%).
c 250 per 1000 (25%).

Discussion

$$\text{The infant mortality rate} = \frac{\text{number of deaths less than a year}}{\text{total number of live births}}$$

$$\text{The neonatal mortality rate} = \frac{\text{number of deaths less than a month}}{\text{total number of live births}}$$

$$\text{The perinatal mortality rate} = \frac{\text{number of stillbirths + first week deaths}}{\text{total number of births}}$$

References
Forfar and Arneil's Textbook of Paediatrics 3–5
Nelson's Textbook of Paediatrics 431–2

ANSWERS

a Diabetes insipidus secondary to trauma. **48**
b DDAVP.

Discussion
Improved management of head injuries has improved the mortality rates post injury. Diabetes insipidus is a rare complication and needs to be differentiated from raised intracranial pressure (causing high blood pressure and bradycardia) or seizures whilst being sedated for ventilation (increased blood pressure, no hypovolaemia).

References
Forfar and Arneil's Textbook of Paediatrics 910, 1110
Nelson's Textbook of Paediatrics 1574–6

---

a 46XX, –14, +t (14 : 21). **49**
b Down's syndrome.

Discussion
A small percentage of cases of Down's syndrome (approximately 5%) are due to a translocation. In most cases, chromosome 21 is translocated onto chromosome 14. The mother has a balanced translocation with 45 chromosomes, whereas her daughter has 46 chromosomes with an unbalanced translocation.

References
Forfar and Arneil's Textbook of Paediatrics 61–2
Nelson's Textbook of Paediatrics 314–5

---

a Aortic coarctation and aortic stenosis. **50**

Discussion
The obvious abnormalities here are massively increased pressure in the left ventricle and increased pressure in the

ascending aorta compared to the descending aorta. Note that the saturations are normal throughout and that she is clinically well. The data fit with a left outflow obstruction, namely aortic stenosis and coarctation.

References
Forfar and Arneil's Textbook of Paediatrics 679–80, 683–4
Nelson's Textbook of Paediatrics 1300–4

51   a Chronic granulomatous disease.
     b His mother.

Discussion
In this condition, phagocytosis occurs but the phagocytic cells are unable to reduce oxygen to hydrogen peroxide. The bacteria are therefore ingested but not killed and may survive within cells provoking a chronic granulomatous reaction and chronic abscess formation.

Diagnosis is made by showing neutrophil liability to reduce NBT, absence of the normal chemiluminescent response of neutrophils at phagocytosis and impaired neutrophil killing. Inheritance of chronic granulomatous disease is usually X-linked although sporadic cases do occur.

References
Forfar and Arneil's Textbook of Paediatrics 1319
Nelson's Textbook of Paediatrics 596–7

52   a 4 and 6 years.

Discussion
In the Goodenough 'draw-a-man' test, the examiner asks the child to draw a man carefully. The child receives one point for each item which is present in the drawing. For each four points, 1 year is added to the basal age which is

3 years. If a child scores eight points, his mental age score is 5 years.

References
The Development of the Young Infant and Young Child (ed. R.S. Illingworth), 9th edn, 1997. Churchill Livingstone, 224

---

a Fructose intolerance.   **53**
b Autosomal recessive.
c Complete avoidance of fructose and sucrose.

Discussion
This baby is hypoglycaemic and has a marked metabolic acidosis. The baby was generally well until she ingested fruit juice, whereupon she became unwell. Hereditary fructose intolerance involves 1-phosphofructaldolase deficiency, therefore fructose 1-phosphate accumulates in the liver and inhibits phosphorylase. This results in transient inhibition of the conversion of glycogen to glucose and therefore hypoglycaemia. Treatment is complete elimination of fructose from the diet.

References
Forfar and Arneil's Textbook of Paediatrics 1206
Nelson's Textbook of Paediatrics 387–8, 427

---

a Kasabach Merritt syndrome with disseminated intra-   **54**
vascular coagulation (DIC).

Discussion
Kasabach Merritt syndrome is the association of thrombocytopenia with vascular tumours. Thrombocytopenia is secondary to entrapment within the lesion and may be followed by DIC. Treatment involves infusions of blood, platelets and fresh frozen plasma. If lesions contain an

ANSWERS

arteriovenous shunt, this may lead to high output cardiac failure. Management options include treatment with steroids, radiotherapy, embolization or treatment with interferon or aminocaproic acid. The latter agents may work by inhibiting proliferation of smooth muscle and endothelial cells.

References
Forfar and Arneil's Textbook of Paediatrics 255, 1696, 1880
Nelson's Textbook of Paediatrics 1431–2, 1839

55
  a Generalized, symmetrical spike and wave complexes at 3 Hz. This is characteristic of petit mal (typical absence epilepsy).

  b Petit mal seizures can be precipitated by hyperventilating, thus if the EEG is relatively normal in a child who has previous clinical features of absence seizures then they can be encouraged to hyperventilate while still recording.

  c The treatment of choice is sodium valproate (80% respond).

Discussion
Absence seizures occur more frequently in boys than girls with a peak incidence at around 6 years. In about a third of cases there is a positive family history. The typical absence seizure lasts for 5–10 s with the child becoming still and staring ahead. They are often first noticed by teachers who think the child is 'day-dreaming'. The attack ends abruptly and the child continues with his or her previous activity. They may occur hundreds of times a day and may be more frequent when the child is tired or hungry.

References
Forfar and Arneil's Textbook of Paediatrics 758–9
Nelson's Textbook of Paediatrics 1688

a Haemolytic uraemic syndrome.   **56**
b Treatment of hyperkalaemia, e.g. with calcium resonium, glucose and insulin or salbutamol.
c Peritoneal dialysis.

Discussion

Haemolytic uraemic syndrome is characterized by micro-angiopathic anaemia, thrombocytopenia and acute renal failure. Most cases occur in infants and young children during summer months and are associated with a prodromal diarrhoeal illness. The more severe type occurs in older children.

Trying to treat individual biochemical or pathological abnormalities here is inappropriate as the underlying problem is acute renal failure. Antihypertensives do not address the underlying fluid overload, diuretics require functioning nephrons and intravenous bicarbonate or plasma exacerbate the hypertension.

Hyperkalaemia may be treated in various ways; calcium resonium rectally will exchange potassium for calcium ions; and intravenous glucose and insulin, and salbutamol promote intracellular movement of potassium.

References
Forfar and Arneil's Textbook of Paediatrics 1064–6
Nelson's Textbook of Paediatrics 1433, 1492–3

a Iron deficiency anaemia.   **57**
b Thalassaemia trait.
c Vitamin D deficiency/rickets.

Discussion

This child's diet puts him at risk of both iron and vitamin D deficiency. Cows' milk and breast milk are both low in these important nutrients.

Thalassaemia trait can present in much the same way (in a similar population) but the ferritin result is normal.

References

Forfar and Arneil's Textbook of Paediatrics 1281
Nelson's Textbook of Paediatrics 146, 1387–8

---

58   a   Transposition of the great arteries.

Discussion

The saturations in the left ventricle and pulmonary artery are the same and the pressures are similar. The pressures and saturations are also very similar between the right ventricle and aorta. This is consistent with two independent circulations which are found in transposition of the great arteries (where the aorta is attached to the right ventricle and the pulmonary artery to the left ventricle). At birth a degree of mixing is allowed by the patent ductus but once this closes the baby quickly becomes hypoxic and cyanosed. Complete closure is incompatible with life. Some babies with this condition have an atrial septal defect or ventricular septal defect which allows some mixing and adequate oxygenation but these infants still require definitive treatment within the first year. The treatment currently offered is arterial switch.

References

Forfar and Arneil's Textbook of Paediatrics 685–90
Nelson's Textbook of Paediatrics 1320–1

---

59   a   ABO incompatibility.

         b   Most cases of ABO incompatibility may be managed with phototherapy; exchange transfusion is rarely required.

Discussion

ABO incompatibility is 5–10 times more common than rhesus incompatibility. It presents in otherwise well term infants in the first 24 h of life. It rarely causes severe problems as most anti-A and anti-B in the mother is IgM and therefore does not cross the placenta. Small quantities of anti-A and anti-B IgG occur but are usually quickly tissue bound by the fetus and therefore sensitization is uncommon. Definite diagnosis depends on identifying anti-A or anti-B antibodies in maternal plasma.

References
Forfar and Arneil's Textbook of Paediatrics 256
Nelson's Textbook of Paediatrics 503–4

60

a Normal exercise test results.
b His symptoms are likely to be related to obesity and weight loss should be recommended.

Discussion

As the exercise test is essentially normal it is likely that his dyspnoea is related to his obesity. Causes of obesity include Prader–Willi syndrome, hypothyroidism and Cushing's syndrome and these may need to be excluded. Other possible causes of breathlessness on exertion include cardiac disease, severe anaemia or other 'organ failure' conditions.

References
Forfar and Arneil's Textbook of Paediatrics 575–6, 1287
Nelson's Textbook of Paediatrics 1177, 1184–5

61

a Marfan's syndrome.
b Homocystinuria.
c Upwards dislocation of the lens.
d Aortic incompetence, mitral valve prolapse.

ANSWERS

Discussion

Marfan's syndrome is inherited in an autosomal dominant fashion. Other features include arachnodactyly, pigeon chest, pectus excavatum, kyphoscoliosis, flat feet, joint hyperextensibility and recurrent dislocations.

Homocystinuria produces a similar clinical picture to Marfan's syndrome except in addition a malar flush and osteoporosis are common and lens dislocation is downwards. There is a high incidence of learning difficulties and those with normal intelligence often have behaviour problems.

Marfan's syndrome is due to an abnormality of mucopolysaccharide metabolism and an excess of hydroxyproline is found in the urine whereas homocystinuria is an abnormality of amino acid metabolism and high levels of homocystine are detected in the urine.

References
Forfar and Arneil's Textbook of Paediatrics 1181–2, 1754, 1756
Nelson's Textbook of Paediatrics 335–8, 1982–3

---

62   a Whooping cough.
   b Pernasal swab.
   c A child may be infectious 7 days after exposure until 3 weeks after the paroxysms begin.

Discussion

Pertussis is a highly contagious condition which is caused by *Bordetella pertussis* and is spread by droplet infection. An irritating cough gradually becomes paroxysmal and may last for 3 months. The typical whoop may not be seen in young infants and apnoeic spells may occur.

The incubation period is 7–10 days and diagnosis is confirmed by culture or immunofluorescence of nasopharyngeal secretions for *B. pertussis*. A white blood count may reveal a lymphocytosis.

Prevention is by immunization as a component of the

primary course of immunization against diphtheria, tetanus and pertussis (DTP), given at 2, 3 and 4 months of age.

References
Forfar and Arneil's Textbook of Paediatrics 636, 1371–3
Nelson's Textbook of Paediatrics 779–83

63

a Transient erythropenia of childhood.
b Bone marrow biopsy to exclude acute lymphoblastic leukaemia.
c The prognosis is good: she should make a spontaneous recovery.

Discussion
In transient erythropenia of childhood there is red cell hypoplasia with a reduced reticulocyte count. The white blood count is normal and the platelet count may be elevated. It may occur following a mild infection and apart from anaemia, examination is unremarkable.

Reference
Nelson's Textbook of Paediatrics 1382

64

a 6–9 months.

Discussion
In a normal baby primitive reflexes appear and disappear at different times and deviation from the expected pattern may suggest a neurological problem. The asymmetric tonic neck reflex is seen in babies in the first 2 months of life. In babies with cerebral palsy it may persist and increase beyond the age of 2–3 months. The grasp reflex diasppears in babies by the age of 2–3 months and the walking reflex by 5–6 months. The Moro response is a vestibular reflex and disappears by 3–4 months of age. The parachute reaction appears at 6–9 months and persists throughout life.

ANSWERS

As this baby has lost the asymmetric tonic neck reflex, the grasp, walking and Moro reflexes, but has not yet developed the parachute reflex, it must be between 6 and 9 months of age.

References
Forfar and Arneil's Textbook of Paediatrics 264
Nelson's Textbook of Paediatrics 1673

---

65 a Hypoxia and a respiratory acidosis.

b Respiratory distress syndrome.

c Other causes of respiratory difficulties in the preterm newborn include pneumonia, pneumothorax, diaphragmatic hernia, heart failure and metabolic acidosis.

Discussion
Respiratory distress syndrome is characterized by tachypnoea, tachycardia, intercostal recession, expiratory grunting and cyanosis.

References
Forfar and Arneil's Textbook of Paediatrics 200–205
Nelson's Textbook of Paediatrics 216, 481

---

66 a Choledochal cyst.

b Ultrasound.

c Excision of the cyst with hepaticojejunostomy.

Discussion
A choledochal cyst is a cystic dilatation of the choledochus. It presents at variable age, sometimes in infancy with obstructive jaundice suggestive of biliary atresia or in the older child with intermittent jaundice, abdominal pain and an abdominal mass.

References

Forfar and Arneil's Textbook of Paediatrics 549, 1870
Nelson's Textbook of Paediatrics 1036, 1119–20, 1152–5

a Cystinuria.   **67**

b Calculus formation causing renal colic, haematuria and
  urinary obstruction with secondary pyelonephritis and
  eventually renal failure.

c A diuresis should be maintained to limit crystallization.
  This may be combined with alkalinization of the urine
  with oral sodium bicarbonate. D-Penicillamine may
  also be given—this chelates cystine to form L-cystine-
  D-penicillamine disulphide which is more soluble than
  cystine and therefore less likely to crystallize.

Discussion

Cystinuria is a disorder of intestinal absorption and renal
tubular reabsorption of cystine, lysine, ornithine and
arginine. Approximately 1 in 600 of the population have
cystinuria but only 3% of those affected form calculi.

References

Forfar and Arneil's Textbook of Paediatrics 1026, 1194
Nelson's Textbook of Paediatrics 1551

a Isoimmune neonatal thrombocytopenic purpura.   **68**

b A transfusion of washed maternal platelets.

Discussion

This condition results from transplacental passage of
maternal specific IgG platelet antibodies as the mother
who is PLA1 negative has made antibodies to her PLA1-
positive infant's platelets. If the infant is given washed
maternal platelets there will be a rapid increase in platelet
count, whereas a normal platelet transfusion produces
only a temporary increase in platelets in the infant, as

the transfused platelets are likely to be PLA1 positive. This situation is analogous to rhesus disease. Intracranial bleeding can be a consequence of this, even *in utero*.

References
Forfar and Arneil's Textbook of Paediatrics 950
Nelson's Textbook of Paediatrics 1434

---

69 Urine turns green in
- phenylketonuria;
- tyrosinaemia;
- histidinaemia.

Urine turns purple with
- salicylates;
- phenothiazines.

Discussion
In tyrosinaemia, histidinaemia and with adrenaline, the urine goes a transient green. In phenlyketonuria it goes emerald green.

Reference
Forfar and Arneil's Textbook of Paediatrics 867–8

---

70 a Williams' syndrome.
b Supravalvular aortic stenosis;
Peripheral pulmonary stenosis.

Discussion
Idiopathic hypercalcaemia associated with learning difficulties, cardiovascular abnormalities and dysmorphic features is known as Williams' syndrome. The characteristic 'elfin face' comprises prominent lips, an upturned nose, prominent cheeks and low set ears. They may develop 'cocktail party chatter' where they learn conversational pieces, which they do not fully comprehend, but

which they can reproduce in social situations giving the impression of language competency.

References
Forfar and Arneil's Textbook of Paediatrics 833
Nelson's Textbook of Paediatrics 318, 475–6, 1611, 1989

71

a X-linked agammaglobulinaemia.
b Intravenous immunoglobulin infused over 2–3 h every 3–4 weeks, depending on clinical response and circulating immunoglobulin levels;
Prophylactic antibiotics.

Discussion
In X-linked agammaglobulinaemia, there is a failure of pre-B cells to mature into functioning B cells. Presentation is with recurrent pyogenic infections, e.g. otitis media, pneumonia, once circulating maternal antibody levels have fallen. Laboratory investigations will reveal reduced levels of immunoglobulins and normal cell-mediated immunity. Circulating lymphocyte markers show a normal T cell pattern with absent B cells, although pre-B cells are found on bone marrow biopsy.

References
Forfar and Arneil's Textbook of Paediatrics 1316
Nelson's Textbook of Paediatrics 567–8, 734–6

72

a Glanzmann's disease.
b Platelet aggregation tests show lack of aggregation with all stimulants (e.g. collagen, thrombin) except ristocetin.
c Autosomal recessive.

Discussion
In Glanzmann's disease, there is a defect of platelet function due to defective formation of ADP storage granules

resulting in a prolonged bleeding time. The bleeding is generally mucosal and may be severe. Specific platelet function tests should be undertaken where there is an elevated bleeding time with normal platelet count and morphology. The next most common recessive disorder is Bernard–Soulier syndrome but here the platelets are enlarged, whereas in Glanzmann's disease the blood film is normal.

References
Forfar and Arneil's Textbook of Paediatrics 254, 950
Nelson's Textbook of Paediatrics 1432

---

73   **a** Truncus arteriosus.
       b DiGeorge syndrome.

Discussion
Both ventricles are at systemic pressure and there is increased saturation in the pulmonary artery. There is a gradual step down through the left side, due to the associated VSD, with the values being equal in the PA and the aorta. These figures are consistent with a single artery trunk arising from the ventricular portion of the heart and supplying the systemic and pulmonary circulation. Truncus arteriosus is seen in patients with DiGeorge syndrome and may be complicated by thymic aplasia, immunodeficiency and hypocalcaemia.

References
Forfar and Arneil's Textbook of Paediatrics 668, 693–4, 1310–1
Nelson's Textbook of Paediatrics 571, 1324–5

---

74   **a** Pseudohypoparathyroidism type 1.
       b X-ray of the hands.
       c Short 4th and 5th metacarpals.

Discussion

Type 1 pseudohypoparathyroidism often presents with symptomatic hypocalcaemia. Other features include variable developmental delay, short stature and obesity. Type 1 is further divided into types 1a and 1b. In 1a there is a reduced level of a protein membrane component coupling the PTH receptor to the catalytic unit of adenylate cyclase, and in type 1b the level is within normal limits. In type 2 there is thought to be an intracellular defect beyond the step of cAMP generation and therefore the response to PTH is normal.

References

Forfar and Arneil's Textbook of Paediatrics 1129–30
Nelson's Textbook of Paediatrics 1608–9

---

a Androgen insensitivity syndrome.   **75**
b Removal of testes;
  Vaginal reconstruction;
  Hormone replacement therapy;
  Psychological support for Laura and her family.

Discussion

Androgen insensitivity syndrome results from the failure of the cells of the mesonephric duct and genital tubercle to respond to circulating testosterone, and therefore male genitalia do not develop. Those affected are phenotypically female but chromosomal analysis reveals 46XY and testosterone levels are in the normal male range. External genitalia appear female but the uterus, fallopian tubes and upper two-thirds of the vagina are absent and presentation may be with primary amenorrhoea. Testes may be found in the abdomen, inguinal canal or vulva and should be removed due to the risk of malignancy.

Chromosomal analysis should be performed to exclude this condition in girls presenting with 'inguinal hernias'.

ANSWERS

References

Forfar and Arneil's Textbook of Paediatrics 1076
Nelson's Textbook of Paediatrics 1644

76

a Risk ratio = $\dfrac{\text{risk exposed}}{\text{risk non-exposed}} = \dfrac{15/2000}{30/8000}$

b Odds ratio = $\dfrac{\text{odds exposed}}{\text{odds non-exposed}} = \dfrac{15/1985}{30/7970}$

c Rate difference = rate exposed – rate non-exposed
$$= 15/3985 - 30/15\,970$$

Discussion

This simple cohort study tests the understanding of risks, odds and rates. It is useful to know that the risk of a disease is the same as cumulative incidence, i.e. the proportion of people in a population who will develop the disease during a particular time frame. The odds of a disease is the probability of getting the disease versus not getting the disease. Both risk ratios and odds ratios are measures of relative risk and tend to be similar values

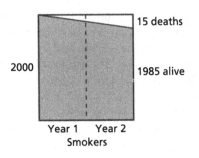

Fig. 17(a)

Person years $(2000 \times 2) - 15 = 3985$
Risk = 15/2000
Odds = 15/1985
Rate = 15/3985

where the risk is small but increasingly different as the incidence of disease increases.

Calculation of the risk ratio and odds ratio is aided by drawing a diagram of the figures in the exposed (Fig. 17a) and non-exposed (Fig. 17b) arms of the cohort.

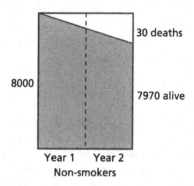

Fig. 17(b)

Person years $(8000 \times 2) - 30 = 15\,970$
Risk $= 30/8000$
Odds $= 30/15\,970$
Rate $= 30/15\,970$

Reference
Basic Epidemiology 29–30, 38, 78

---

a Autosomal recessive.   **77**
b 1/2.
c 1/2.
d $1/2 \times 1/2 \times 1/4 = 1/16$.

Discussion
Cosanguinity increases the risk of a child being affected with an autosomal recessive condition, as there is an increased chance of both parents carrying the defective gene. In this case both (a) and her partner (b) have a 1 in 2 chance of being carriers. The risk of (c) being affected is the risk of his parents × 1/4 (autosomal recessive).

References
Forfar and Arneil's Textbook of Paediatrics 72–3
Nelson's Textbook of Paediatrics 309

---

78 a Sickle cell anaemia.
   b Target cells, poikilocytes, Howell Jolly bodies and sickle cells.
   c Haemoglobin electrophoresis which will show HbS (90–95%), HbF (5–10%);
       Sickle test.

Discussion

Sickle cell anaemia is a disorder of haemoglobin synthesis due to a single amino acid substitution (valine for glutamine) in the beta-globin chain. It usually presents at over 6 months of age when HbF (alpha2, gamma2) levels have fallen. Presentation is usually with dactylitis, anaemia, icterus and hepatosplenomegaly. Repeated splenic infarction results in less prominent splenomegaly in older children. Due to splenic dysfunction there is an increased risk of infections, for example, pneumococcal infections and salmonella osteomyelitis.

Painful crises can occur due to vaso-occlusion, causing severe pain in the abdomen, muscles and bones. These crises should be treated with analgesia and adequate hydration. Urine and blood cultures should be performed and a throat swab sent. Broad spectrum antibiotics should be given.

Anaemic crises result from marrow aplasia, megaloblastic crisis and visceral sequestration of red cells or haemolysis. Whole blood transfusions are indicated for severe crises.

References
Forfar and Arneil's Textbook of Paediatrics 931–4, 1325
Nelson's Textbook of Paediatrics 1396–1400

ANSWERS

a Abnormal activity in right hemisphere leads only. This indicates a focal abnormality.

b Space-occupying lesions such as tumours and abscesses may give such a pattern.

c CT scan or MRI scan.

79

Discussion

Headaches in children occur for a variety of reasons. There may be raised intracranial pressure, the headaches may be vascular in origin, they may be a manifestation of a systemic illness or they may be psychogenic in origin. Indications for imaging include localizing signs, persistent visual disturbance, early morning headaches, deterioration in school performance or marked behavioural change and headaches associated with seizures. An abnormal EEG pattern as shown here is also an indication for further imaging, e.g. CT or MRI scan. An MRI scan provides better images of posterior fossa structures and gives better definition of infiltrating tumours.

References

Forfar and Arneil's Textbook of Paediatrics 782–3, 970–1
Nelson's Textbook of Paediatrics 1704–5, 1731–4

---

a Renal vein thrombosis.

b Ultrasound.

c Treatment is supportive—attention to fluid balance and correction of electrolyte abnormalities.

80

Discussion

Renal vein thrombosis is associated with the hypercoagulability which accompanies hyperosmolar dehydration, asphyxia, polycythaemia and nephrotic syndrome. It is also more common in infants of diabetic mothers.

Presentation is usually with haematuria, an enlarged kidney and thrombocytopenia. There is often evidence of

ANSWERS

intravascular coagulation such as elevated fibrin degradation products or consumption coagulopathy. If renal vein thrombosis is bilateral, renal failure may occur and management options include heparin therapy or thrombectomy.

References
Forfar and Arneil's Textbook of Paediatrics 287, 1066
Nelson's Textbook of Paediatrics 436–7, 1494

---

81 a This is fluorescent in-situ hybridization technique (FISH).
b This illustrates a chromosome 22 deletion.
c DiGeorge syndrome and Shprintzen syndromes.

Discussion
The detection system has a built-in control, that is a second probe which hybridizes to the tip of the long arm. Thus the normal 22 has both the control signal and the DiGeorge region signal (close to the centromere) while the deleted 22 has only the control signal 0.

References
Forfar and Arneil's Textbook of Paediatrics 1305
Nelson's Textbook of Paediatrics 571, 1606

---

82 a 2.5–3.0 years.

Discussion
A child should be able to build a tower of 6–7 bricks and draw in a circular scribble at 22–23 months. Most know their sex by the age of 2 1/2. Copying a circle usually comes by the end of year 3 and bridge building in year 4.

References
Forfar and Arneil's Textbook of Paediatrics 451–2
Griffiths Mental Development Scales

ANSWERS

a Nephrotic syndrome.

b Infection—peritonitis is the most frequent type of infection, with *Streptococcus pneumoniae* being the most common organism involved;
Thrombosis—both arterial and venous occur.
c 'No added salt' diet;
Fluid restriction;
Steroids.

Discussion

Nephrotic syndrome occurs when proteinuria results in hypoproteinaemia and oedema. Boys are more commonly affected than girls, with a peak incidence at 1–5 years of age. The majority of cases are idiopathic but it may occur secondary to a variety of conditions including Henoch–Schonlein purpura, malaria or renal vein thrombosis. Oedema is the usual presenting feature and there may be ascites and pleural effusions. Hypovolaemia may result in abdominal pain and peripheral ischaemia and infarction. Nephrotic syndrome is a hypercoagulable state with increased levels of fibrinogen and reduced levels of antithrombin III.

Minimal change nephrotic syndrome is usually steroid responsive and prednisolone ($60\,mg/m^2/24\,h$) should be given daily in divided doses until the urine has been protein free for 3–5 days. Alternate day single-dose therapy should then be given for at least a further 28 days. If there are repeated relapses despite treatment with steroids then cyclophosphamide therapy should be considered.

References

Forfar and Arneil's Textbook of Paediatrics 1057–61
Nelson's Textbook of Paediatrics 1500–3, 1513

a Hepatitis B virus is present in high concentrations in

ANSWERS

blood, serum and serous exudates, therefore midwives need to take extreme care to avoid contamination at the time of delivery.

b The baby should have specific immunoglobulin (HBIG) and three doses of hepatitis B vaccine. The first dose should be given within 12 h of birth, with further doses at 1 month and 6 months of age.

c Mothers with hepatitis B can breast feed providing the baby is immunized at birth.

Discussion

Hepatitis B is transmitted parenterally, sexually and by perinatal transmission from mother to child. Those carriers in whom e-antigen (HBeAg) is detected are the most infectious. Babies born to such mothers should therefore be given HBIG as well as three doses of hepatitis B vaccine. Those with antibody to HBeAg (anti-HBe) are generally of lesser infectivity and should receive active immunization only.

References

Forfar and Arneil's Textbook of Paediatrics 315–6
Nelson's Textbook of Paediatrics 911–2
Roberton's Textbook of Neonatology 1012

85　a Thalassaemia;
Haemoglobinopathies, e.g. sickle cell disease, HbC, HbSC;
Iron deficiency anaemia;
Post-splenectomy;
Liver disease;
Severe dehydration.

Discussion

Target cells are erythrocytes which on staining have a well-stained central area, then an intermediate pale zone and a well-stained periphery. They are thinner than normal and have an increased resistance to hypotonic saline.

a Turner's syndrome;
   Noonan's syndrome.
b Turner's syndrome = coarctation of the aorta;
   Noonan's syndrome = pulmonary stenosis and HOCM.

Discussion

In Turner's syndrome lymphoedema with redundant skin at the back of the neck may be noted at birth. In childhood, features include short stature, webbed neck, widely spaced nipples and a low posterior hairline. At puberty there may be a failure of development of secondary sexual characteristics and primary amenorrhoea. Renal anomalies are common including duplex ureters and horseshoe kidneys.

Features of Noonan's syndrome include short stature, hypogonadism, hypertelorism, ptosis, epicanthic folds, low-set ears, pectus carnatum or pectus excavatum, cubitum valgum and neck webbing.

References

Forfar and Arneil's Textbook of Paediatrics 67–68, 435–439
Nelson's Textbook of Paediatrics 1630, 1635–7

a Acute lymphoblastic leukaemia (ALL).
b Poor prognostic features include
   • white blood count > $50 \times 10^9/l$ at presentation;
   • CNS disease at presentation;
   • age < 2 years or > 10 years at presentation;
   • T cell type;
   • chromosomal abnormalities, e.g. translocations;
   • massive mediastinal widening.

Discussion

Leukaemia is the commonest childhood malignancy with ALL accounting for 75% of cases. The peak age of presentation is at 2–6 years, and the male : female ratio is

1.2 : 1. Presenting symptoms include fatigue, pallor, infections, lymphadenopathy and bone pain. Cranial nerve palsies indicate central nervous system involvement. If leukaemia is suspected, the following investigations should be performed — full blood count and film, bone marrow biopsy, cytogenetic studies, lumbar puncture, blood culture, chest X-ray, urea and electrolytes, creatinine, calcium, phosphate and urate.

References

Forfar and Arneil's Textbook of Paediatrics 942–4
Nelson's Textbook of Paediatrics 1453–5

88 a Surgical debridement of the wound;
　Reinforcing dose of adsorbed tetanus vaccine;
　Human tetanus immunoglobulin;
　Penicillin.

Discussion

As he has not had the recommended 5-dose tetanus regimen as he has not yet had his school leavers' vaccine, he should therefore receive a reinforcing dose of adsorbed tetanus vaccine. He also needs a reinforcing dose of low-dose diphtheria vaccine and polio vaccine. As he has a tetanus-prone wound (a puncture wound), he should also receive a dose of human tetanus immunoglobulin.

References

Forfar and Arneil's Textbook of Paediatrics 382–4
Nelson's Textbook of Paediatrics 815–7, 1017

89 a Chediak–Higashi syndrome.
　b Severe pyogenic infections;
　Lymphoproliferative syndrome.

Discussion

This is a rare autosomal recessive disorder which is characterized by partial albinism and abnormal neutrophil granulation. Severe pyogenic infections occur and later hepatosplenomegaly and lymphadenopathy with thrombocytopenia which may be fatal.

References

Forfar and Arneil's Textbook of Paediatrics 1307, 1320
Nelson's Textbook of Paediatrics 594–5

90

a Atrial septal defect.
b Cardiomegaly with an enlarged right atrium; Increased pulmonary vascularity.
c Surgical closure.

Discussion

The main abnormality is an increase in saturation between the vena cava and the right atrium. All other values are within normal range. This is consistent with an atrial septal defect. If the defect is not closed, right-sided overload and failure may occur.

References

Forfar and Arneil's Textbook of Paediatrics 674–5
Nelson's Textbook of Paediatrics 1288–92

91

a A booster dose of diphtheria, tetanus and polio is required but a booster dose of pertussis is not recommended.
b No, as the incidence of invasive disease with *Haemophilus influenzae* type b falls sharply after the age of 4 years, routine immunization of children over 4 and adults is not recommended.
c He should have two doses of mumps, measles and rubella (MMR) vaccine given 3 months apart.

ANSWERS

Discussion

The current immunization schedule recommended in this country is:

BCG	given to high risk infants
Hepatitis B	given to high risk infants
DTP, Hib and polio	1st dose 2 months 2nd dose 3 months 3rd dose 4 months
MMR first dose	12–15 months
Booster DT and polio	3–5 years
MMR 2nd dose	3–5 years
BCG	10–14 years or infancy
Booster dT and polio	13–18 years

References

Forfar and Arneil's Textbook of Paediatrics 383
Nelson's Textbook of Paediatrics 1015–6

---

92   a Red cell galactose 1-phosphate uridyl transferase level.
       b Galactosaemia.
       c Galactose and lactose-free diet.

Discussion

Galactosaemia is due to a deficiency of galactose 1-phosphate uridyl transferase which enables galactose to be converted to glucose. It is inherited in an autosomal recessive fashion. Symptoms occur once feeding is established, and breast-fed babies are more severely affected due to the higher lactose content in breast milk. Symptoms include diarrhoea and vomiting, failure to thrive and prolonged jaundice. Anaemia, clotting abnormalities, hepatosplenomegaly, hypoglycaemic convulsions and cataracts may also occur. Long-term treatment consists of a strict lactose and galactose-free diet with expert dietary advice. If not treated, mental retardation, behaviour problems, progressive cataracts, liver and renal damage may occur. With good dietary control normal development should be possible.

References

Forfar and Arneil's Textbook of Paediatrics 324, 1205–6
Nelson's Textbook of Paediatrics 386–7

93

a Phaeochromocytoma.
b Measurement of plasma catecholamine levels;
Tumour localization by ultrasound, CT or isotope scanning.

Discussion

Phaeochromocytomas are catecholamine-secreting tumours and are a rare cause of secondary hypertension in children. Although the tumours usually arise in the adrenal glands, they may occur anywhere in the sympathetic chain. They may be associated with multiple endocrine neoplasia (MEN) types 1 or 2, or neurofibromatosis. Hypertension may be sustained or paroxysmal. Less than 10% of tumours are malignant but once identified the tumour should be removed. Depending on the catecholamines produced by the tumour, alpha or beta blockade may be required prior to surgery.

References

Forfar and Arneil's Textbook of Paediatrics 1143
Nelson's Textbook of Paediatrics 1370, 1626–8

94

a Central diabetes insipidus.
b DDAVP plus careful attention to fluid balance.

Discussion

This baby has developed diabetes insipidus following

ANSWERS

meningitis. There is inadequate secretion of ADH from the hypothalamus, resulting in the production of a large volume of dilute urine due to failure to concentrate it. As there is not a compensatory increase in oral intake, hypernatraemic dehydration results. Treatment is with synthetic ADH (DDAVP) given intranasally.

References
Forfar and Arneil's Textbook of Paediatrics 1110–1
Nelson's Textbook of Paediatrics 1574–6

---

95 a 100%.
 b 2/3 (66.7%).
 c $1/20 \times 2/3 \times 1/4 = 1/120$.

Discussion
Cystic fibrosis is an autosomal recessive condition. It occurs in a person whose parents both carry recessive genes, thus (a) must be a carrier. Following simple Mendelian theory, (b) has a two-thirds chance of carrying the gene. The chance of offspring having cystic fibrosis is the population risk (i.e. father's risk) × mother's carrier risk × 1/4 (autosomal recessive inheritance).

References
Forfar and Arneil's Textbook of Paediatrics 626–8
Nelson's Textbook of Paediatrics 309

---

96 a Feto-maternal haemorrhage.

Discussion
The diagnosis is unlikely to be isoimmune haemolytic anaemia as the mother and baby have the same blood group, and the Coombs test is negative. A positive Kleihauer test identifies fetal haemoglobin in the maternal circulation, confirming feto-maternal haemorrhage.

References
Forfar and Arneil's Textbook of Paediatrics 248
Nelson's Textbook of Paediatrics 499

---

a Clinitest tablets are based on the Benedict's test and will   **97**
   detect reducing substances in the urine.
   Substances which test positive with clinitest tablets include:
   - glucose;
   - fructose;
   - galactose;
   - lactose;
   - sucrose;
   - pentose;
   - vitamin C;
   - homogenistic acid.
b Clinistix are specific for glucose.
c Galactosaemia.

Discussion
If the clinitest result is positive, further chromatography
may be done to determine which substance is present.
The most likely diagnosis in this boy is galactosaemia.
Although severe cases present soon after birth, presentation may be delayed in milder cases, children presenting
with poor feeding, poor weight gain and cataracts.

References
Forfar and Arneil's Textbook of Paediatrics 867, 1205
Nelson's Textbook of Paediatrics 386–7

---

a Colour of stools and urine, family history, whether there   **98**
   is hepatosplenomegaly.
b Hepato-biliary scintigraphy (99m-Tc-iminodiacetic
   acid) — IDA;
   Ultrasound;
   Alpha-1-antitrypsin levels.

ANSWERS

c Extra-hepatic biliary atresia;
   Alpha-1-antitrypsin deficiency.

Discussion

This baby has obstructive jaundice. As the TORCH screen and hepatitis screen are negative and the urine is negative for reducing substances, the main differential diagnosis is alpha-1-antitrypsin deficiency and extrahepatic biliary atresia. In extrahepatic biliary atresia there is prolonged conjugated hyperbilirubinaemia with complete stool pallor. An ultrasound may show increased intrahepatic parenchymal echoes and an IDA scan will show good uptake but no tracer in the bowel over a 24-h period. Diagnostic tests should be performed as soon as possible if biliary atresia is suspected as a delay in treatment will adversely affect prognosis. The treatment of choice is Kasai's hepatic portoenterostomy.

Alpha-1-antitrypsin deficiency may present in the neonatal period with cholestasis which needs to be differentiated from biliary atresia. The diagnosis is made by assay with electrophoresis to identify the precise genotype. There are numerous variants with >90% of the normal population being homozygous PiM. It is those who are homozygous PiZ who develop neonatal cholestasis.

References

Forfar and Arneil's Textbook of Paediatrics 244–5, 651, 1250, 1863–4
Nelson's Textbook of Paediatrics 495–6, 1135–6

99 a Supraventricular tachycardia (SVT).
   b Vagal stimulation (facial immersion in cold water for 10 s);
     Intravenous adenosine (50 µg/kg initially, 100 µg/kg if no improvement);
     D.C. conversion;
     Flecanide, amiodarone, sotolol, propranolol and digoxin are also used in some centres.

ANSWERS

Discussion

SVT is the most common abnormal tachycardia in children and most do not have underlying congenital heart disease. In infancy SVT may be associated with tachypnoea and pallor, and if the episode is prolonged (> 24 h), cardiorespiratory distress may occur. Older children may complain of feeling faint, of having a fast heart rate or more rarely they may experience chest pain. Clinical examination between episodes of SVT is unremarkable. During an episode of SVT the ECG has a regular rate of 220–300 beats/min, with 1 : 1 atrioventricular conduction.

References

Forfar and Arneil's Textbook of Paediatrics 226, 697
Nelson's Textbook of Paediatrics 1339–40

---

a Post-streptococcal glomerulonephritis.

100

b Pyelonephritis.
c Treatment is not usually required but strict attention to fluid balance is required to minimize the chance of fluid overload.
d 95% of children make a complete recovery following post-streptococcal glomerulonephritis and further attacks are infrequent.

ANSWERS

Discussion

Post-streptococcal glomerulonephritis typically occurs 7–14 days after a group A beta-haemolytic streptococcus throat infection but may follow other streptococcal infections. It usually affects school age children. Investigations reveal gross haematuria with variable proteinuria, and minimal to severe renal failure. The C3 and C4 levels may be reduced during the acute phase but return to normal levels after approximately 8 weeks.

Ninety-five per cent of children make a complete recovery following post-streptococcal glomerulonephritis and further attacks are infrequent. Renal function usually returns to normal within 10–14 days but microscopic haematuria may persist for 1–2 years. Antihypertensives may be required if hypertension is not controlled by fluid restriction.

References

Forfar and Arneil's Textbook of Paediatrics 1047, 1049–53
Nelson's Textbook of Paediatrics 1487–8

---

101 a Constitutional delay in growth and puberty.
b Final adult height may not be reached until around 20 years of age but should be appropriate for the parental target height range.
c None.

Discussion

In this condition children are 'slow maturers'. Height and bone age are usually delayed by 2–4 years and the onset of pubertal maturation is also delayed, corresponding to the child's bone age. Often there is a family history of this condition. Sexual development, although delayed, is normal. No further investigations are necessary but reassurance is required.

References

Forfar and Arneil's Textbook of Paediatrics 433–4
Nelson's Textbook of Paediatrics 1572

---

102 a Transdermal fluid losses causing hypernatraemic dehydration.
b Urine and serum osmolality.
c Pay strict attention to fluid balance;
Increase local humidity by creating a humidified microenvironment.

Discussion

The transdermal fluid loss is dependent upon ambient temperature and humidity and is increased by phototherapy and nursing babies in open incubators. Transdermal losses are greater in premature babies, particularly soon after birth. This is partly due to a poorly developed horny layer of the epidermis, and as the stratum corneum matures over the first weeks, the transdermal losses decrease. It is essential that strict attention is paid to fluid balance in the premature infant, with monitoring of urea and electrolyte levels.

References

Forfar and Arneil's Textbook of Paediatrics 163, 481–2
Nelson's Textbook of Paediatrics 207

103

a Increased QT interval of approximately 0.45 s.
b Jervell–Lange–Neilsen.
c Romano–Ward.

Discussion

The normal QT interval is less than 0.4 s. A prolonged QT interval is found in Jervell–Lange–Neilsen where it is associated with ventricular arrhythmias and congenital hearing loss. A prolonged QT interval is also found in Romano–Ward syndrome. Hypocalcaemia and hypokalaemia may also give rise to a prolonged QT interval. In hypokalaemia there may be a U wave at the end of the T wave.

References

Forfar and Arneil's Textbook of Paediatrics 698
Nelson's Textbook of Paediatrics 1273–4

104

a 17-Hydroxyprogesterone level.
b Congenital adrenal hyperplasia (CAH).

ANSWERS

c This condition is life threatening unless treated promptly — the baby should be resuscitated and hydrocortisone and fludrocortisone (a mineralocorticoid) given. Replacement therapy needs to be lifelong.

Discussion

The baby is profoundly hyponatraemic with a milder degree of hypochloraemia and hyperkalaemia. The clinical picture fits with a diagnosis of congenital adrenal hyperplasia where there is a disorder of adrenal steroidogenesis and thus a deficiency of cortisol. The most common disorder is 21-hydroxylase deficiency (95%), but 11β hydroxylase and 3β hydroxysteroid dehydrogenase may also be deficient. In the classic 21-hydroxylase deficiency form, the plasma levels of 17-hydroxyprogesterone are markedly elevated and the blood cortisol levels are low.

CAH may be salt losing or non-salt losing, and this baby obviously has the more severe salt-losing type.

References
Forfar and Arneil's Textbook of Paediatrics 1134–8
Nelson's Textbook of Paediatrics 1617–22

---

105 a A banded karyotype illustrating a female trisomy 13.
b Microcephaly, midline scalp defects, low-set ears, polydactyly, flexion deformity of the fingers, single umbilical artery and cryptorchidism.

Discussion

Trisomy 13 (Patau's syndrome) has an incidence of about 0.07 per 1000 live births. Most cases are due to non-disjunction. Infants usually survive only a few days or weeks.

References
Forfar and Arneil's Textbook of Paediatrics 64–5
Nelson's Textbook of Paediatrics 314–6

a McCune–Albright syndrome. **106**
b Skeletal survey.

Discussion

In this condition there is an association of hyper-pigmented macules, precocious puberty and thinning and sclerosis of the bones. Precocious puberty is the usual presentation and vaginal bleeding is a common early feature. There are associated multiple endocrinopathies with glandular hyperfunction giving rise to e.g. Cushing's syndrome, thyrotoxicosis, hyperparathyroidism and hyperprolactinaemia.

References

Forfar and Arneil's Textbook of Paediatrics 430–1
Nelson's Textbook of Paediatrics 1584–5

a Pulmonary stenosis and ventricular septal defect. **107**
b Tetralogy of Fallot.
c Surgery is the definitive treatment. There may be a one stage repair or a palliative procedure prior to the total repair. In a classical Blalock–Taussig operation the subclavian artery is transected and anastomosed to the pulmonary artery, or in the modified procedure there is insertion of a Goretex graft between the two.

Discussion

The saturations are low throughout the right side and also in the left ventricle and the aorta. The step down from the left atrium to the ventricle indicates some mixing of arterial and venous blood, i.e. via a ventricular septal defect. The pressure in the right ventricle is markedly elevated but normal in the pulmonary artery; this is consistent with pulmonary stenosis. Combining these data with the history of cyanosis in an infant the most likely diagnosis is tetralogy of Fallot. It may be possible to do one-stage corrective surgery or several operations may be required. The prognosis following surgery is good with most individuals leading a 'normal' life.

References
Forfar and Arneil's Textbook of Paediatrics 688–90
Nelson's Textbook of Paediatrics 1311–5

---

108   a Toxocara infection.
b Toxocara ELISA test.
c Diethylcarbamazine or thiabendazole;
Steroids for ocular lesions.

Discussion
The natural hosts of *Toxocara canis* are dogs and foxes. Children ingest eggs from soil which is contaminated with dogs faeces or they ingest eggs directly from the animals themselves. The larvae penetrate the bowel wall and then proceed to involve other organs including the liver, lungs, heart, kidneys or eye. There are two distinct forms of toxocaral infection: generalized toxocaris associated with eosinophilia and ocular toxocaral disease.

In the generalized form, investigations reveal eosinophilia and elevated immunoglobulin levels, particularly IgM, IgG and IgE. The toxocara ELISA test is the most reliable serological test with a biopsy required to make a definitive diagnosis.

Treatment is with diethylcarbamazine or thiabendazole, and steroids may be required for ocular lesions. Regular worming of dogs is important and dogs should be encouraged not to defecate in areas where children play. Children should learn the importance of hand washing after handling pets.

References
Forfar and Arneil's Textbook of Paediatrics 1541–4, 1757
Nelson's Textbook of Paediatrics 1004–5

a Neurosensory hearing impairment.

109

b Genetic or secondary to an intrauterine infection, e.g. cytomegalovirus (CMV) infection.

Discussion

Sensorineural deafness may be secondary or acquired. Deafness may be inherited in an autosomal dominant or recessive fashion, or it may be X-linked. It may be associated with various syndromes including Treacher–Collins syndrome, Pendred's syndrome or Usher's syndrome. Other cases of congenital deafness may be secondary to teratogenic drug ingestion in pregnancy or intrauterine infection, e.g. CMV, rubella, toxoplasmosis.

Acquired causes of sensorineural deafness may be secondary to infection, e.g. meningitis, mumps, asphyxia, hyperbilirubinaemia, treatment with otoxic drugs, or associated with neurodegenerative or neurocutaneous disorders.

References

Forfar and Arneil's Textbook of Paediatrics 844–5
Nelson's Textbook of Paediatrics 1806

a This EEG illustrates centro-temporal spikes and spike-waves. This is typical of benign rolandic epilepsy.

110

b The prognosis is excellent, seizures often stopping around the age of 12 years.

c Treatment with carbamazepine or valproate is usually effective.

Discussion

This form of epilepsy is the most common partial motor epilepsy in childhood, typically occurring in young children 4–10 years of age, with a higher incidence in boys. Seizures usually involve paraesthesia of one side of the face with or without tonic–clonic movements of this side of the face. Nocturnal generalized tonic–clonic fits sometimes follow.

References

Forfar and Arneil's Textbook of Paediatrics 762–3
Nelson's Textbook of Paediatrics 1688

---

111 a Turner's syndrome.

b Karyotype. This should have been done before anterior pituitary function tests were considered.

Discussion

This case illustrates a case of primary ovarian failure associated with short stature. The FSH and LH are abnormally high throughout. Turner's syndrome has a frequency of 1 in 5000 and commonly presents as failure to thrive or primary amenorrhoea.

Serum oestrogen, buccal smear and pelvic ultrasound are other investigations which may be performed but would not give a definitive diagnosis. If growth hormone is used in girls with Turner's syndrome their final height may be increased by several centimetres.

References

Forfar and Arneil's Textbook of Paediatrics 67–8, 435–7, 1077
Nelson's Textbook of Paediatrics 317–8, 1573, 1635–6

---

112 a Daunorubicin cardiomyopathy.

b Serial echocardiography.

Discussion

Daunorubicin is a drug widely used to treat acute leukaemias, lymphomas and solid tumours. Common side-effects include nausea and vomiting, myelosuppression and alopecia. High cumulative doses are associated with the development of a cardiomyopathy and total cumulative doses should be limited. Sequential radionuclide ejection fraction measurement may assist in safely limiting total dosage. If symptoms of congestive cardiac failure develop the prognosis is poor.

References

Forfar and Arneil's Textbook of Paediatrics 943–4
Nelson's Textbook of Paediatrics 1351
British National Formulary, edn 35, March 1998. BMA / Royal Pharmaceutical Association

---

a Cytomegalovirus (CMV) infection.   **113**

b Hearing tests;
   Ophthalmology review;
   Measurement of CMV antibody levels.

Discussion

CMV is the most common congenital infection. About 50% of females of childbearing age will be susceptible to CMV infection in pregnancy. The incidence of congenital infection is 3–4/1000 births but 90% of these will be asymptomatic in the newborn period. Those who are symptomatic show the classical signs of intrauterine infection — low birthweight, hepatosplenomegaly, rash and septicaemia. Those who are symptomatic often show sequelae — microcephaly, chorioretinitis, deafness and learning difficulties. Diagnosis in the newborn period is relatively easy, raised IgA in cord blood or IgM in neonatal blood being diagnostic. The virus may be isolated from saliva or from urine and typical inclusion bodies are seen in cell deposits of fresh urine.

References

Forfar and Arneil's Textbook of Paediatrics 315, 1420–1
Nelson's Textbook of Paediatrics 523, 895–7

---

a *Listeria monocytogenes* pneumonia.   **114**

b Resuscitation and intravenous ampicillin plus an aminoglycoside.

c This condition has a high mortality.
d Whether microabscesses were seen in the placenta.

Discussion

Listeria monocytogenes is a non-spore-forming Gram-positive bacillus which may cause a mild flu-like illness if infection occurs during pregnancy. It may result in abortion, stillbirth or premature delivery. Microabscesses, skin granulomas, enlarged liver and spleen and the passage of meconium in a preterm infant are suggestive of *Listeria* infection. Pneumonia in the affected infant is very common, and the mortality rate is greater than 30% despite treatment with ampicillin combined with an aminoglycoside. Diagnosis is confirmed by culture of the organism and ELISA testing.

References
Forfar and Arneil's Textbook of Paediatrics 312
Nelson's Textbook of Paediatrics 810–1

---

115 a Urine for microscopy and culture.
b To cut down on her feeds.

Discussion

It is essential to take a clear history to establish if the baby is truly vomiting and not regurgitating food as occurs in gastro-oesophageal reflux. Vomiting may occur in intestinal obstruction (bile may be present), pyloric stenosis (projectile vomiting), metabolic disorders or infections. If the baby looks well and clinical examination is normal, it is important to exclude a urinary tract infection and to look at her feeding pattern, checking that her bottles are being made up correctly. This baby is getting 220 ml/kg of milk and is probably vomiting as she is being overfed.

References
Forfar and Arneil's Textbook of Paediatrics 502
Nelson's Textbook of Paediatrics 1033

ANSWERS

INDEX

140